A
Crisis of Meaning

12/11/96

To My friend ~~Bob~~ Bob,
with affection &
appreciation

Love
Stn

A
Crisis of Meaning

How Gay Men Are
Making Sense of AIDS

Steven Schwartzberg

New York   Oxford
Oxford University Press   1996

Oxford University Press

Oxford   New York

Athens   Auckland   Bangkok   Bogotá   Bombay
Buenos Aires   Calcutta   Cape Town   Dar es Salaam
Delhi   Florence   Hong Kong   Istanbul   Karachi
Kuala Lumpur   Madras   Madrid   Melbourne
Mexico City   Nairobi   Paris   Singapore
Taipei   Tokyo   Toronto

and associated companies in
Berlin   Ibadan

Published by Oxford University Press, Inc.
198 Madison Avenue, New York, New York 10016

Library of Congress Cataloging-in-Publication Data
Schwartzberg, Steven
A Crisis of Meaning : How Gay Men Are Making Sense of AIDS /
Steven Schwartzberg.   p. cm.   Includes index.
ISBN 0-19-509627-4
I. AIDS (Disease)—Psychological aspects.   2. Gay men—Diseases.
3. Adjustments (Psychology)   I. Title.
RC607.A26S377   1996
362.1'858682'0086642—dc20   96-11004

"The Thistle, The Nettle" from *Provinces: Poems 1987–1991* by Czeslaw Milosz. Copyright
1991 by Czeslaw Milosz Royalties, Inc. First published by The Ecco Press in 1991.
Reprinted by permission.

"The Thistle, The Nettle" reprinted by permission of Sterling Lord Literistic, Inc. Copyright
1991 Czeslaw Milosz.

"Diagnosis" and "I dreamed" from *Lingering in a Silk Shirt* by Walta Borawski. Copyright
1994 by Walta Borawski. Published by Fag Rag Books in 1994. Reprinted by permission.

1 3 5 7 9 8 6 4 2

Printed in the United States of America
on acid-free paper

In loving memory of Gregory

Diagnosis

When the doctor and the tests
confirm you are ill begin

to learn to breathe. Hold on to
a crystal your lover or your

god. Watch your favorite
tv shows read books

that teach or make you laugh
escape or go deeper Don't

smoke cigarettes or drink
alcohol; Take vitamins, eat

good food, keep working and
exercise Don't curse fate or

spend energy wishing things
were otherwise They're not

Today is still yours
Be good to it

Walta Borawski

Preface

*W*riting about AIDS and life's mean-
ing may seem a misbegotten enterprise. Words cannot compete with an
epidemic. Language falls short of the mark. What phrases could capture
the courage, the accomplishments, the horror, the grief? With AIDS, words
do not elucidate the truth but diminish it.

Yet words must be attempted—to heal, to encourage, to offer solace or
refuge, to bear witness. And to stab at meaning amid the chaos. For even in
the face of great sorrow, the struggle for a meaningful life need not be
abandoned. The world continues on. So do our personal journeys for
meaning, individually and collectively.

In this book, I present a psychological perspective for how gay men
(particularly HIV-positive gay men) have found ways to live meaningfully
amid HIV and AIDS. My aim is to chronicle this defining feature of modern gay culture—the remarkable transformations some men have accomplished, the anguish of meaninglessness that weighs others down, the vapor
of grief that hangs in the air.

I start with a few basic premises: To find (and maintain) meaning in life
is a fundamental human need. The greatest psychological threat of HIV, or
any trauma of such magnitude, is how it can destroy meaning. And all of
us have the ability to grow, to deepen our life's meaning, no matter our circumstances or current functioning.

If any meaning is to be found amid tragedies such as AIDS, perhaps it
only emerges through learning to accept paradox. Sorrow and joy, growth
and loss, suffering and healing, living and dying—each is tied most to the
thing it seems to resemble least. In a world turned upside down, accepting

the essential union of opposites may offer a possible pathway to stability, change, and growth.

Yet even with this said, life's meaning can never be laid out in a tidy fashion, like so many ducks in a row. It contains mysteries beyond our ken. And psychology is a young upstart in mapping this domain—theology, mysticism, the arts, philosophy, and science can all stake a rightful shared claim to the territory. Psychology offers but one sliver of understanding.

And so I am wary of much that psychological research tells us about the human condition, and encourage readers to share my wariness. Having studied research methodology, I fret at how easy it is to manufacture results that sparkle numerically but misrepresent human experience. How comforting the false illusion that we can know and chart that which is amorphous, daunting, and larger than ourselves!

It is in this spirit that I offer the thoughts of this book—cautiously, admittedly subjectively, the clinician in me more ardent than the researcher. And although I believe (and hope) the journeys of meaning I present will speak to many people's experience, they are not meant to be a perfect or complete map. Major differences lie between any theoretical framework and the unique details of each life.

I will portray individual lives, but I also speak of "gay men," the "gay community." These, too, are imprecise. Gay men's lives vary tremendously, influenced by matters of race, cultural background, economics, and the host of social, political, and personal forces that shape identity. Throughout, I try to strike a balance between the specific and the general, between what characterizes a particular person and what shades into us all.

I also write aware of HIV's devastating impact globally. Gay men in Western cultures are but one part—and, in the context of AIDS worldwide, a minor part—of this epidemic. The impact and pain of HIV extend far beyond the confines of any one community or subculture.

The lives of nineteen men living with HIV figure prominently in the book. In my descriptions of these men, I have taken care to protect their confidentiality. All names, and other key pieces of identifying information, have been changed, but in all cases I have attempted to maintain the tenor and gist of their words. For readers interested in keeping track of these men as they appear throughout the book, a list is provided for this purpose in Appendix A.

The men I interviewed for this project have left an indelible impression on me. Their poignant words, their humanity and courage, have affected how I live, how I approach psychotherapy, how I think of life and death. By entrusting me as they did with their stories, I feel some sense of moral urging to provide a legacy for them, to keep a part of them alive. I feel this as a fellow gay man, as a fellow human, and as a privileged invited witness to their pains, triumphs, and fears.

"Gently they go, the beautiful, the tender, the kind. Quietly they go, the intelligent, the witty, the brave. I know. But I do not approve. And I am not resigned."[1] Adversity has much to teach us about living meaningfully. To write about AIDS is to fall short of the mark. Not to write about it is to abandon hope.

Cambridge, Massachusetts   S.S.
March 1996

Acknowledgments

I wish to acknowledge, with great appreciation, the contributions of many people who helped bring this work to fruition. Michael Bronski, James Levi, Dr. Jill McAnulty, Dr. Larry Rosenberg, Dr. Robert Schoenberg, and Dr. Michael Seiver read the book in draft form and provided wise guidance on honing a final manuscript. Joan Bossert was an enthusiastic and astute editor, and Jed Mattes a fine literary agent and strong advocate for the project. Thanks also to Rosemary Wellner for her attentive copy editing.

For their support, friendship, encouragement, advice, love, enthusiasm, or help with specific information, I thank Jay Blotcher, Kevin Cathcart, Dr. Jack Foehl, Dr. Donna Fromberg, Dr. Paula Fuchs, Becky Johnson, Dr. Melanie Katzman, Dr. Ken Mayer, Michael Owings, Dr. Richard Schwartz, Dr. Joseph Shay (for the metaphor of movies and photos), and Steve Wilson. Drs. Richard Halgin and Ronnie Janoff-Bulman were inspiring teachers—the book is inextricably tied to their encouragement and support.

I am tremendously appreciative of the 19 men who participated in the research interviews that form the base of this work. Positive Directions generously assisted with locating willing participants. Sigma Xi, the Scientific Research Society, partially funded the original interview study with a grant-in-aid of research.

Finally, my parents, Marilyn and Nat Schwartzberg, have always provided gifts that I try not to take for granted—love, acceptance, and, by example, a model for facing unexpected sorrow with resilience and courage.

Contents

I'm hopeful that as more and more people are living longer and longer with AIDS and as HIV-positive, that we'll start talking about not just what's keeping these people alive and healthy, but also about the good things that it's brought out in us as a people. We are teachers, we are bridges, we can find ways. Gay people have always found ways to survive and to be ourselves. You can go back into history and find we've always been there. . . . Whitman said, "I perceive one picking me out by secret and divine sign."

Craig

I've taken part in some of the most incredible of the social experiments of the twentieth century, with great pleasure, and I would say I am totally unrepentant. I've learned a lot. . . . We may have to wait a generation or two before people are ready to pick up and take a look at a lot of the stuff that's happened, but that's not unusual.

Ron

I couldn't have written this, I don't think anybody could have thought this up. If anyone had thought it up or written it, and people read it, they would have said it's too fantastical, it's impossible that this kind of stuff could happen: people don't have lives like this, people don't do these things, people don't have these things happen to them.

Victor

I've heard, and this might be my fantasy, that at the cathedral at St. John the Divine, the crucifix that dominates the apse is a columbarium, a relic or container of ashes of the dead. I've heard that it's mostly a container of ashes of people who have died of AIDS, and I love the idea that if I die, my ashes could go there and be part of that cross with other gay people. I like the idea of being buried with other victims of this epidemic. I don't want us to be forgotten as individuals or as a community who went through some spectacular suffering.

Anthony

HIV is my blessing—I thank God he gave me this blessing to help me grow.

Francis

Part One

Introduction

1

A Crisis of Meaning

*I*n June 1981, the weekly newsletter of the Centers for Disease Control noted an unusual medical occurrence. In the previous six months, five young gay men in Los Angeles had all been diagnosed with *Pneumocystis carinii* pneumonia (PCP)—a rare disease, virtually unseen in young American men. Two had died. The blurb ran on the newsletter's second page, followed by a long article on alcohol consumption in Utah.

Nothing akin to the Los Angeles oddity was mentioned again for several weeks. But slowly, new and equally puzzling reports dribbled in. From New York City: twenty cases of Kaposi's sarcoma, a rare skin cancer, usually found in elderly men of Mediterranean descent. From Los Angeles: six more cases of Kaposi's, and a few new ones of PCP. From San Francisco: Kaposi's sarcoma, PCP, and a smattering of other unusual maladies. Within one year, the CDC accumulated over 350 of these increasingly alarming reports. Six months later the number topped 1,000— almost all fatal, almost all among otherwise healthy gay men.[1] Unnamed, mysterious, and unlike anything previously seen, the impossible seemed to be happening. An awful and fierce epidemic was taking shape.

A page-two blurb, an unnamed oddity—it's hard to imagine that such a relatively short time ago, something so fundamental about modern life, modern gay life, just didn't matter. AIDS was simply not part of the picture. It wasn't there to ravage us. It wasn't there to mock and invalidate some of the most basic, if unconscious, beliefs by which we had come to guide our late twentieth-century lives. It wasn't there to rob us of our lovers, our friends, our acquaintances, our lives. To weaken us. Or to strengthen us.

AIDS has altered the very fabric of gay men's private and communal lives. The change has been cataclysmic—a seismic jolt off the Richter scale of psychological earthquakes. So much of what once could be taken for granted no longer can; so much of what mattered no longer does. Old beliefs about how the world works are no longer viable. Old assumptions about life are no longer true. AIDS has changed everything.

On any measure, by any scale, this is a tragedy of great magnitude. For those living with HIV and those intimately affected by it, the disease is an omnipresent reality, infiltrating, seeping into most every cranny of day-to-day existence.

The psychological challenges posed by the epidemic are enormous. For gay men, a slew of harsh demands now press on our lives with unremitting insistence. We have had to learn, and must keep learning anew, how to grieve individual, multiple, ever-accumulating deaths. We have been forced to develop new strategies to cope with enormous, previously unforeseen, obstacles: maintaining vigilant safety with sex, facing a cultural stigma greater even than homophobia, acclimating to life in a world soaked in loss. We have had to forge ways of balancing grim reality with soothing, necessary hope.

We have struggled, privately and publicly, to maintain a capacity for optimism—even joy—while daily life may be tinged with a pain never completely out of awareness. We have wearily attempted to juggle mammoth, seemingly incompatible tasks: mourning the dead, tending the ill, protecting the healthy.

These are great challenges indeed.

Yet with adversity as daunting as that posed by the epidemic, one psychological challenge rises to a place of paramount importance. This challenge surpasses, and encompasses, all the others. It is at the root of survival (psychological, and perhaps physical) in this era. The challenge: how to establish, or recreate, a life of meaning in the face of such potentially overwhelming trauma.

AIDS is much more than a health crisis. For gay men, it has unleashed a crisis of meaning. With so much loss and grief in its wake, so many lives affected in wrenching and unexpected ways, AIDS has obliterated many people's prior beliefs of the world as meaningful. In its enormity, intensity, and relentlessness, AIDS cuts to the very heart of how people find meaning in life, of how to understand the world and our place in it.

We have been thrust into a world where profound issues—mortality, fate, spirituality, dying, the purpose of living—no longer hide politely, diplomatically out of daily awareness. These are no longer luxuries of idle philosophic indulgence. They press with an urgency that demands our reluctant attention.

In the best of times, exploring how we create a life of meaning can be a personal inquiry of helpful benefit. In times of massive crisis and potentially unremitting sorrow, it is a psychological task of fundamental importance.

———————————

This assault on some of our most basic, core beliefs leads to several crucial questions. How, if at all, do gay men—and especially those among us living with HIV—make sense of AIDS? Is finding meaning in AIDS really important? Are there things a person can do to facilitate this process?

The answer to the first question is complex—much of the rest of this book is dedicated to answering it. The answers to the second and third questions are each a hearty, if qualified, "yes." In brief, what I present in this book is a psychological framework for how HIV-positive gay men have (and have not) found meaning in HIV and AIDS. Living with HIV is often a life journey into an unknown world, a frightening psychological voyage into *terra incognita*. With the ideas I offer here, I hope to provide a new map to help people locate, understand, and perhaps steer a course in that journey.

The terrain I survey reveals oases of strength and growth, as much part of the topography as tragedy and pain. This is dismal land, from which all would surely leave if they could. Yet to emphasize *only* the horror of HIV belies the testimony of too many people who know otherwise from rugged experience. This paradox of the epidemic cannot be denied: Against the bleak backdrop of pain that surrounds us, some folks have developed a capacity to savor life that they previously did not, or could not, know.

The terrain is vast, each individual's journey unique. How varied the routes, how different the challenges: a 19-year-old boy in rural Colorado with no gay friends, infected by an older partner who assured him of his safety; a 40-year-old New Yorker, once enraptured with the jubilant atmosphere of the late 1970s, now ill and bereft of his large social circle; a divorced man, coming out late in life, grappling with the inescapable irony of how embracing life led to facing death. For each person with HIV the paths of meaning vary, shaped by personal experience and the trappings of one's world.

Still, all with HIV inhabit the same land and need to chart a course. People undertake this struggle for meaning with a variety of attitudes, strategies, and degrees of deliberateness. Some embrace the search as a rallying point for more passionate living. Others yearn for meaning but cannot find it, becoming mired in a quest marked by self-defeat, futility, and embitterment. Still others regard the challenge to meaning as a surprisingly unimportant undertaking (often to the disbelief of onlookers). Some scale heights, others flounder. Most meander through, at first blindly, learning more as they go.

The journey of reclaiming meaning may be a major preoccupation, or only an incidental sliver of a person's experience. It may be embraced or feared. The scope is wide, but the issue fundamental: it is in the realm of life's meaning that HIV insists upon its greatest psychological recompense.

Most people have an oddly morbid penchant for remembering bad news, and many gay men can tell you when they first heard of AIDS—the first rumor or gossip, the first news report or unsettling obituary, the first sudden, unexpected illness of a friend or acquaintance.

Yet more accurately, for most of us—especially those who participated in pre-AIDS gay culture—accepting the unbelievable fact of AIDS' existence happened gradually. In the early 1980s we heard about it bit by bit, over time, in ragged pieces. We greeted the news with some personal mixture of confusion, disbelief, illusory arrogance, denial, and fear. What was it, who gets it, how could this be?

But at a certain point it became real. Perhaps suddenly. AIDS took on an actual face, a body, a name. It stopped being an abstraction, and metamorphosed into a horrible reality. A dying friend. An ill lover. A positive test result.

For me, AIDS became real in July 1984. My friend Robby Beck was diagnosed. Robby was 24 years old, waif-like, earthy, funny, street-savvy. This was early enough in the epidemic that it was still shocking to actually know someone diagnosed with AIDS, to have it hit so close to home (at least in Philadelphia, where I lived at the time). HIV was not yet matter-of-fact. I recall realizing that although I *had* previously assumed AIDS was real, it wasn't—not to me. Robby was somewhere about the 1,600th case documented in the United States. For me, he was case Number One. The first face of AIDS in my life.

Each of us has our own Robby, our own Case Number One. Many of us now have too many faces and names, too many Robbies, to bother counting.

The process of Robby's illness and dying was memorable. It was painful, of course, and exhausting, and frightening. But something extraordinary happened through the roller-coaster course of his disease. A circle of dedicated friends came together to take care of him. We were young. Most were unaccustomed to being in the presence of such severe illness—or coping with anything quite so serious.

So much had to be learned: how to face and overcome our automatic fears, in order to tap an inner strength previously dormant. How to maintain, and communicate, hope. How to empty bedpans, remove soiled sheets, change diapers. How to tolerate breathing in the sharp and often repugnant odors of a deteriorating body. How to comfort Robby, and each other. How to decide when to encourage him to fight, when to let go.

As Robby's health worsened, the community around him strengthened. Without purposely setting out to do so, together we created something far greater than any of us had anticipated, or signed up for: we participated— caringly, respectfully—in someone's death. We transformed and eased the harshness of Robby's dying by embedding it in a community of love. Love was what we all felt—for Robby, from him, for each other.

Robby died in April 1985. Those who shared in taking care of him mourned his loss. Yet we also took away what felt like a precious gift. Somehow we were innocent no more, and far less young. It was a terrible, sad, eye-opening rite of passage. AIDS was undeniably real. We had experienced its pain. We had railed against its utter unfairness and lack of justice. And we had glimpsed the paradox of extreme tragedy: In Robby's dying, each of us found a place of love and spirituality in ourselves, or the universe, or both, we had not known before.

Robby's dying has not left me. It has been tempered and colored by many other deaths, the passage of time, the relentless tenacity of AIDS.

Nor was Robby's death my first brush with grief: My only brother died of acute-onset leukemia when we were both teenagers, decimating the tranquility of an otherwise uneventful suburban upbringing.

Perhaps my brother's death, unexpected and jarring, first implanted within me the personal importance of struggling with meaning; his dying had a monumental impact on my adolescence. But as a quirk of fate particular to my life, I came to see his death not just as a grievous loss, but as a sad foreshadowing of what was soon to follow. My brother's death clearly exerted its influence, yet the legacy of Robby's journey with AIDS seems to have had the more transformative effect, and to solidify for me one enduring question: How do people find meaning in life, amid the hardship and tragedy of major trauma?

As the AIDS toll has inexorably amassed, the question has grown ever more central. How can one make sense of the widely differing responses to HIV reflected in the gay community? Where is the meaning, for me, for others?

I recall the experience, a few years back, of attending a gay pride march in New York City. At such events, I divide my time between joining the parade and staying on the sidelines, watching the marchers and the passersby. I happened to be sitting on the curb when the dense throngs of the AIDS groups marched by. The vast range of what HIV has triggered in us was, quite literally, paraded before me.

A large spiritual group led the way. One hundred or so strong, they filled the air with lovely, beatific chanting and the seductive clatter of finger-cymbals and tambourines. On their heels ran ACT-UP, storming more than marching up the avenue, impassioned and energized with the justness of their cause. In stark contrast, a cadre of solemn, silent men followed next. They held haunting poster-sized photos of once smiling friends and lovers.

The groups continued on, as if the parade might never end. Each blew by with its own energy, each a fierce new wind in a chaotic hurricane. Volunteer caregivers and buddies, long-term survivors, political lobbyists, people with AIDS self-help organizations, folks in recovery, hospice workers, Friday Night supper clubs. Every color, every race, every age.

In the groups, the marchers, the crowd, how could I make sense of the dizzying array of what I saw around me? Where is the meaning, for me, for others?

I saw men with empty, frightened eyes—men in whom AIDS had destroyed a capacity for hope and vitality. Yet others positively beamed—men for whom HIV seemed to unlock a newfound ability to celebrate life. In some, I saw the dangerous allure of "quick-fix" solutions: the shallow, feel-good, "I-can-have-complete-control-over-my-body-by-thinking-good-thoughts" response. Still others radiated a razor-sharp anger—an anger admirably honed in battle against an inept and homophobic government, yet impotent in fighting fate's larger and indifferent cruelty.

And I saw, more than anything else, a grief beyond measure or words. A stunning, numbing, bewildering, soul-wrenching, unspeakable grief.

Where is the meaning, for me, for others?

I believe that this disparate range of responses can be understood from one unifying vantage point: the crisis of meaning AIDS has produced. More than there being a "right" or "wrong" way to respond to the epidemic, the private and communal responses of gay men to HIV can be seen as reflecting this crucial challenge—sometimes frantic, sometimes agonizing, never easy—of how to unearth, or create, meaning from what life has become.

With the ideas of this book, I attempt to describe this landscape of meaning, to make sense of what I see when I look at the lives of those who have been touched by HIV. I realize the haughtiness and foolishness of this task. Words are paltry and inadequate with a challenge so deep, a trauma so large. Yet I also believe that words and ideas, however incomplete or flawed, can make a difference.

I write from the perspective of three converging strands in my life.

First, I write as a clinical psychologist. In psychotherapy, I am continually struck by how the search for meaning—even a hunger for meaning—is crucial in people's lives and struggles. This is of course true with such issues as HIV, which challenge our mortality. But this search extends far beyond, and constitutes one of the basic needs (some would even say drives) that make up the human condition.

One of my patients was a promising research scientist whose career (and much the rest of her "normal" life) was abruptly derailed by the late onset of a severe, chronic schizophrenic illness. She has been left unable to meet the demands of typical adulthood—yet remains jarringly aware of all she has lost. Another has never recovered from a single catastrophic event that reshaped his life: watching from the sidewalk, helplessly, as his wife was struck and killed by a hit-and-run driver. Still another is a middle-aged woman whose entire adult life has been marred by the insidious destructive legacy of childhood sexual abuse. For them, as well as for many others, the unspoken focus of their pain is the need to see meaning in their lot, and the inability to do so.

Second, I write as a researcher. To learn more about these questions of AIDS and meaning, I conducted a series of clinical research interviews with HIV-positive gay men. Over the course of the winter and spring of 1990-1991, I met with 19 seropositive gay men. Three questions guided my underlying intent, and my express purpose, in approaching these interviews: How, if at all, have HIV-positive gay men found meaning in, or made sense of, AIDS? How do people, faced with such major adversity, maintain or re-create the belief in a meaningful world, even as external reality has been so dramatically altered? How has AIDS affected HIV-positive gay men's beliefs about such issues as fate, religion, death, the meaning or purpose of life, and the degree to which people control their own destiny?*

The men I spoke with were between 27 and 50 years old. They had known of their HIV infection for between 18 months and nine years.[2] Most had not experienced any HIV-related health impairments, but several had some health difficulties, most commonly fatigue or weight loss. In a few cases, these health difficulties had begun to interfere with daily functioning. None of the men had AIDS, by the criteria then in use; today, several would carry an AIDS diagnosis because of a T-cell count below 200.

Perhaps everyone has a story to tell and privately yearns to tell it. That is what the interviews felt like: men eager to offer their stories, their wisdom. Through them, I witnessed an incredibly rich and varied panoply of the ways HIV had entered into and shaped people's lives (and how people had shaped HIV in their lives). I am not a physician, and have limited knowledge of things medical. Yet with the interviews I felt as if I had been granted use of a valuable stethoscope, with which I could listen in on the inner workings of people's minds and hearts—and gain information as relevant to their lives as CD4 lymphocyte counts and blood plasma levels.

This study is described in detail in Appendix B.

With candor, insight, eagerness, and a remarkable ability to share of themselves, the men spoke eloquently about how HIV had affected their views of the world, their senses of themselves, and how they lived their lives. Throughout this book, I interweave their stories as examples of the different styles and strategies I describe. These men have responded in different ways to their own infection and AIDS' impact in the gay community. Each has his own personal style of coping, his own victories and defeats in finding (or not finding) meaning in his situation.

And third, I write as a gay man. What an extraordinary era it has been for gay people to live in—a time of unprecedented empowerment, of making ourselves proudly visible and known; a time of unprecedented sorrow, of bearing an ever-deepening grief. In the losses I have suffered, the strengths I have discovered, the life choices I have made, and the emotional currents that swirl within, these two predominant drifts of the current era perhaps overshadow all else in shaping who I am, how I live. How I relish—and would fiercely protect—the luxury I am afforded of choosing to live openly as a gay man. How profoundly my life has been marked by living in a culture now wearily acclimated to loss, mourning, and the melancholy awareness of how fragile everything can be.

AIDS is not the only event with the power to destroy life's meaning. From other major adversities we can find half-parallels, half-truths to shed light on what we now live through—comparisons that both edify and obscure.

For example, AIDS bears many similarities to other severe illnesses, such as cancer. Yet it is different from most other illnesses in its communal nature: AIDS attacks the individual *and* the community. People with cancer don't live in a world where many of their friends and neighbors also have cancer. Nor do most people who are ill (at least in Western cultures) carry with them the heavy toll of lethal infectiousness—one of the prime psychological burdens of living with HIV.

In other ways, AIDS parallels a natural disaster. Its most devastating effects have reverberated through select neighborhoods and communities, and it struck with a suddenness that took everyone off guard. Like an earthquake or tidal wave, it leaves massive destruction in its wake. Yet it differs from natural disaster in its ongoing, cumulative nature. AIDS did not happen once and then end. It is not over. It plows inexorably on. Gay men and other besieged communities have not yet been afforded the potential for healing, or meaning, that can come with closure, moving on, or the curative passage of time. Our death watch wearily continues.

In other ways, AIDS parallels war and holocaust. In the sheer enormity of death and bereavement, in the chaotic upheaval of regular life, in its utter inversion of life's ground rules, AIDS has bombarded us with the devastation of wartime. It is a trauma of epic proportion. But again it differs, for it is not, presumably, an intentionally inflicted, malevolent, human-wrought atrocity. Nor is it like life in a concentration camp or amid genocidal terror, where immersion into sadistic deprivation is complete and inescapable.

Severe illness, natural disaster, war: each of these captures an aspect of gay men's lives with HIV. Each offers instruction for us, but each falls short. Some things we can learn from other tragedies. Others we must forge anew.

Another feature unique to AIDS is the virus's slow progression.[3] Today, people living with HIV often know of their infection for a long time, years perhaps, while outwardly maintaining robust physical health. This long waiting period—a grey zone of health and nonhealth, of HIV's simultaneous invisibility and omnipresence—is a time of uncertainty linked with dread linked with hope. There are no clear timelines, no guarantees about the future. This is life in a psychological incubator. Some men use this time to incubate hope, strength, and wisdom. Others, despair and defeat.

———————————

The framework that I offer is straightforward. Of the various lenses we can use to gain a perspective on human experience, I believe the lens of life's meaning is apt to be particularly relevant in understanding gay men's reactions to HIV and AIDS. By way of prelude, four main points deserve special mention.

First, many gay men have successfully forged meaning out of the impact of HIV and AIDS in the gay community—and among those who haven't, many have the capacity to do so. This process of meaning-making is continuous, with no end point, no set fixed destination. It can sail smoothly ahead, or move in fits and starts. It is not a "stage" process; it does not proceed in predictable steps on a marked course. And it is a journey where many of the more prominent signposts may be misleading, faded, or just plain wrong.

Second, although no two individuals go about it in quite the same way, some common patterns typify how people find meaning in HIV and AIDS. As the men I interviewed told me about their lives, ten main themes resounded over and over again. I came to think of these themes as the ways in which people subconsciously understand or organize their own life's journey—the stories or yarns we mentally spin for ourselves. I call these themes "representations" of HIV and AIDS.

These representations vary in how sound or adaptive they are. Some offer refuge and shelter. Others are ill equipped to keep out chill winds of despair, sorrow, and hopelessness. They serve as building blocks of meaning. In varying combinations and to different degrees, these representations shape how people find or maintain meaning in the face of AIDS. We will explore them in detail in Chapter 3.

Third, beyond these representations, people vary in their overall adaptation to life with HIV. I describe four styles of adaptation: Transformation, Rupture, Camouflage, and Impassivity.

In *Transformation*, a person successfully converts the challenges of HIV into a fuller appreciation of life. Men with this style demonstrate vitality, personal growth, emotional stability, and hope—yet they may also experience a sorrowful awareness of loss.

Rupture describes men whose lives have been shattered by AIDS. These men are devastated by loss—actual deaths, and the loss of life's meaning. Men with this style tend to experience significant depression, anxiety, bitterness, feelings of disempowerment, and fear.

Camouflage is the style of men who show a tenuous integration of HIV into a new framework for life's meaning. These men are struggling, perhaps successfully, to stay afloat. But the emotional trauma of HIV may exceed their ability to cope, and they hide their true pains and fears from themselves and others. A potential danger of this style is that when our inner framework for meaning hinges too greatly on self-deception, it can leave us especially vulnerable to difficulty in hard times.

And then there are those who demonstrate a style of *Impassivity*. These men seem surprisingly indifferent to the impact of HIV and AIDS. This minimal reaction may be unrealistic or potentially harmful—yet it can also be a psychologically sound way of dealing with major upheaval if it does not interfere with responsible self-care.

These styles are abstractions, patterns that speak more to general trends than to the rich detail of individual lives. As I describe them more fully in

Chapters 4 through 7, I will include portrayals of men who typify each response. The men's lives are real, replete with accomplishment, imperfection, foibles, and courage.

Finally, with no guarantee of success, there are ways to facilitate the process of rebuilding meaning in life. Few things are as impressive (and mysterious) as the resilience of the human spirit, and I have witnessed people emerge from the ravages of despair to a reinvigorated capacity to cherish life. In Chapter 9, I offer suggestions for people living with HIV to further their journey. Yet I also offer a crucial word of caution: Do not expect in these pages an active self-help book, a "how-to" guide for living with HIV.

I offer nothing akin to "seven easy steps to a life of meaning with HIV." To do so, I believe, would be fraudulent—yet another of the misleading signposts too commonly found in response to the enormity of the challenges. Misrepresenting this journey as simple or straightforward insults and disparages its seriousness, and belittles the remarkable feats that many have accomplished.

Any recovering addict can assure you that "Just say no" to drugs offers little sustained guidance for sobriety. Similarly, "Just say yes" to finding meaning in HIV mocks the reality of the struggle. Most often, no prior experience in a person's life matches the emotional intensity of accepting the reality of HIV. To pretend otherwise would be hokum.

Wonderful things have been accomplished: major new starts in life, quiet moments of small but absolute triumph. Yet prescribing these changes, alas, often does not work. Much of the journey must be self-discovered rather than dictated. So while I offer suggestions that may facilitate the process of integrating HIV into a life of meaning, be forewarned: this is not a primer on turning trauma into triumph.

No, not a primer, but a map—or a looking glass. I describe what I see as the psychological realities of how HIV affects life's meaning, as mirrored in gay men's lives. The lens through which we look cannot help altering what we see. I offer these ideas as a new lens, a new set of lenses.

My hope is that people struggling with HIV—in themselves, in others—may see themselves reflected somewhere in the words and life stories of this book, and come away with a fresh angle for self-understanding—with the possibility of growth, comfort, or validation emerging from this new line of vision. I imagine the response to these ideas not to be,

"Here are the things I should do," but more, "Yes, *this* is what I have felt. This is where I have been. This is where I hope to go."

From one vantage point, the world I describe is quite specific: I speak about the successes and struggles of gay men who live with HIV. These are the life journeys I attempt to plot. The words of HIV-positive gay men bring these concepts to life. Yet this book is written for others as well— gay men who are HIV-negative or uncertain of their antibody status, friends and family members of people with HIV, seropositive individuals from all communities, psychotherapists, and the many men and women whose lives have been reshaped by this epidemic.

Within the gay community, it is not only those living with HIV who struggle with AIDS' enormous impact. Many seronegative gay men have also been touched by the horror and pain. You do not have to be infected to be ensnared in the grief that AIDS has visited on our communities. To survive, witness, or live through an ongoing atrocity such as AIDS leaves its own mark.

For gay men (and others) who are affected but not infected, who are immersed in the epidemic at home or in their community, the challenges to life's meaning are real and deserving of respect. Life's meaning can easily be shattered, or resurrected, for all whose lives have been altered by this epidemic.

Similarly, all people living with HIV, regardless of how they contracted the virus, share many of the same burdens, fears, and challenges. The context and surroundings of illness may differ, but the virus follows the same course. The microbe itself knows not if its host is a white gay man, a Latina woman, a child in Kansas City, or an intravenous drug user in Hoboken.[4] Some basic aspects of living with HIV differ based on a person's situation—whether you belong to a community where HIV is prevalent, or how public judgment of "innocence" or "guilt" fuels a self-perception of stigma.[5] These differences are of course important. Yet much remains similar: All people with HIV need to make sense of a potentially overwhelming trauma and to face the challenge of recreating meaning in life.

I also write for psychotherapists who work with people affected by HIV and AIDS. To such individuals on the "front lines" of the epidemic,[6] I offer these ideas as an alternative template for understanding the psychological impact of life amid an ongoing crisis. And I ask that psychotherapists temporarily hold in abeyance much of what is, in less extreme circumstances, of great value in our current understanding of psychological functioning.

In these pages I do not speak the language of contemporary diagnosis. I seldom refer to disorders of mood, anxiety, or personality, to neurosis or delusion, to tasks of self-efficacy or cognitive restructuring—all of which may apply. I do not describe the men from the vantage point of object relations theory or self-psychology, as I might in my own clinical practice. Instead, I present an alternative view for how people strive to rebuild a world of meaning amid severe crisis. Our current knowledge of psychological functioning is rich, varied, and deserving of great respect; yet with challenges as great as recreating a life of meaning amid massive upheaval, standard models fail and leave us wanting.

Further, although this book is specifically about living with HIV, much of what I say may also apply to living with other struggles, other adversities. AIDS is a massive trauma to incorporate into life—and yet, it is only one trauma, one difficulty among many. Lives are touched by adversity in a slew of ways: severe illness or disabling accident, interpersonal violence, unexpected sorrows or tragedies. Amid *any* trauma, a primary task of coping (and healing) is learning to rediscover or re-create meaning in life.

Reading this book is apt not to be a dispassionate experience. Nor should it be. Some passages may ignite a sense of inspiration or admiration—I convey tales of quietly heroic triumph. But some are apt to be mournfully sad, for an accurate portrayal of life with HIV must give due credence to the grief and sorrow. Other passages may be angering or enraging—anger at the injustice and bewilderment of it all, or perhaps because in my own subjective vision, I miss something important.

I encourage you to approach these ideas with an open mind, without pre-set expectations. If you are reading to help map your own life, it may be of most benefit to sift through the various traits and styles I describe without forcing yourself into a rapid self-definition or categorization. Most likely, you will identify with some points, dismiss others, and feel challenged by still others. Don't jump to conclusions too quickly, for some of what you read may be personally relevant—and helpful in an ongoing journey of growth—but at first feel uncomfortable or disquieting. Approached this way, the book may offer a fresh way of understanding your inner experiences regarding HIV and AIDS.

Many aspects of AIDS medical treatment have evolved significantly since the time of these interviews. AZT is no longer the sole, or most effective, weapon in our arsenal. T-cell counts no longer offer the most sophisticated measurement of HIV's damage. Cycles of medical optimism and pessimism wax and wane. Yet the search for meaning transcends the details of the day. Our crisis of meaning is as relevant now fifteen years into the epidemic as it was at five, or will be at twenty — regardless of whatever encouragements or disappointments science may hold in store.

And so to set the course for where we will go, let us first travel elsewhere. Much of relevance to people's struggle for meaning amid AIDS can be gleaned from what others have discovered about this most basic of human challenges—in times of catastrophic upheaval, and in the quiet, absolute importance of each person's life. If life's meaning is indeed a little-explored but crucial psychological terrain, let us see how other cartographers have made sense of this ambiguous, important territory.

2

Meaning: The Perennial Quest

Not long ago, I had the opportunity to meet with Daniel, a 22-year-old man finishing his senior year of college. Despite the trappings of a well-to-do suburban upbringing, Daniel's life had been marked by extraordinary stress. His parents divorced, acrimoniously, when he was 11 years old, and then he was orphaned at the age of 17. In a morbid coincidence, both his parents died within months of each other, each from an unrelated illness. His siblings (a small horde of half and step brothers and sisters) were engaged in a bitter feud over what remained of the estate — most of which seemed to be withering away through legal fees. At 22, Daniel had already faced losses and life stresses typical of someone well beyond his years.

Yet given these difficult events, Daniel was doing quite well. He was successfully graduating from college, had a circle of good friends, and still maintained a sense of youthful, genuine buoyancy. Despite all that life had hurled his way, Daniel was still able to muster a necessary optimism to face his circumstances.

How did Daniel find meaning in the life events that had befallen him? We will return to his story shortly to see how he made sense of his travails. But before looking more closely at Daniel, and at the tribulations of HIV, let us examine some more mundane circumstances. How do people create meaning in ordinary, everyday life?

The Best of Times:
How Life's Meaning Unfolds in Daily Life

On an everyday basis, we rely on a network of unconscious beliefs to make sense of our lives and our place in the world. These beliefs can be regarded as the infrastructure of life's meaning. Rarely seen or examined, they provide crucial support and definition.

For most people, most of the time, these underlying beliefs work quite well (or at least well enough). They help us feel the world is safe, orderly, and knowable. They give us enough security to venture out with reasonable expectations of what we will find. These beliefs are an unseen screen through which we filter incoming information—a means to comprehend, organize, and respond to the incredible amount of stimulation that bombards us. They provide a rhyme and reason to our days.

We typically stitch together life's meaning from many small threads, from the gradual accrual of seemingly minor details. The few moments of crucial decision and fateful chance impact that burst into each of our lives seldom define its course. Such moments may have great immediate effect. But like bright comets shooting through the night, their glow soon fades and the sky returns to its previous display.

No two people create life's meaning in quite the same way. Each person's construction is unique, shaped by a wealth of personal experience, early family environment, and the vagaries of life. This cumulative sum of experience, along with biological aspects of temperament or resilience, results for each of us in a narrative of life's meaning that defies replication.

Yet despite these individual differences, we also have much in common. How we seek meaning in life is tethered by some deep-seated cultural assumptions. In fact, the similarities between people are as noteworthy as the differences. Many of our fundamental beliefs are shared, jointly molded by culture.

These cultural assumptions are often considered so basic, so matter-of-fact, that they typically go completely unexamined. And even more than this, we often do not regard them as matters of relative opinion: we hold them as absolute truths. Yet many of our deepest beliefs about life and the world are quite subjective—and easily shattered when unmasked as the illusions they really are.

What are some of these core beliefs, so basic to how we create meaning in life, at least in Western cultures? Some help us make sense of the world, others aid us in understanding ourselves.

Psychologist Roy Baumeister theorizes that people base their life's meaning in four central domains.[1] First is a sense of purpose. We want our lives to have some larger goal, some function or rationale, some role in the greater scheme of things. For many people, this sense of purpose is synonymous with meaning: If my life has a purpose, then it has meaning. Second is a sense of value, or morality. People adopt a code of ethics by which we judge our own (and others') actions. Meaning comes from upholding, perpetuating, or staying true to a moral framework. Third is efficacy. We desire to be effective and capable, in control of our lives. To live meaningfully is to be the master of our own fate. And fourth is a sense of self-worth. We derive meaning in life from believing we are deserving, worthy, decent human beings.

For Baumeister, people look to each of these domains, to some degree, to find meaning in life. Shortcomings in one area may lead to overemphasizing another. However people concoct their own personal mixture of meaning, Baumeister thinks that purpose, value, efficacy, and self-worth are its primary ingredients.

Approaching the same concepts somewhat differently, psychologist Ronnie Janoff-Bulman argues that a small number of specific core beliefs influence how most people create life's meaning. Growing from her extensive work with traumatized individuals, Janoff-Bulman notes that most people in Western cultures share the following core beliefs about the meaning of life: (1) the universe is just and fair; (2) people can (and should) control the outcome what happens to them; and (3) life events are not distributed randomly, but follow the rules of cause and effect.[2]

Let's look at these in more detail, on an everyday basis, and in lives now shaped by HIV.

First, justice. Most of us assume that an abstract sense of justice is the guiding principle of the cosmos. We bemoan when something "isn't fair" —implying, of course, that things *should* be fair, that fairness or justice is the principle on which the world ought to be based. Each of us may assign the source of this fairness differently—perhaps we imagine it determined by God, or fate, or nature. Whatever the particular source, we tend to believe that we live in a world governed by ultimate justice.

We also extend this belief in justice to how we view people. We see, or look for, justice in a person's life—a connection between a person's character and what happens to him or her. The universe is not only just, we assume, but this justice is based on morality, and individual lives should reflect this basic abstract law of moral justice.

In other words, good and bad life events are not distributed randomly or by chance: People get what they deserve. If you're a good person, good things will happen to you. If you're bad, you'll be punished.

We apply this rule to ourselves as well. When good things happen, we often take it as confirmation of our goodness or worthiness—"Finally! I deserve this!" When bad things happen, we wonder: What did I do wrong? For what sin or crime am I being punished? What did I do to deserve this? (Some people turn this rule upside down. Good events in my life are undeserved, negative events confirm that I deserve to be punished. This inversion often results from fragile self-esteem—yet observe how a powerful underlying belief in justice still holds sway.)

This unconscious belief has been called the "just world hypothesis."[3] We assume the universe is, or should be, fair and moral. Bad things shouldn't happen to good people.

We also grant the same prominence to a belief in personal control. In Western cultures, and perhaps particularly America, we place extreme value on people's ability to steer their own destinies. We believe people have the ability to control their fate. We take this even further: People have the responsibility to do so.

Along with justice, this is one of our most cherished cultural notions, and one of the most basic underpinnings with which many people build their life's meaning. We tend to believe that people can, and should, control the course of their lives by exerting proper effort. By engaging in the right behaviors, and working hard enough, a person will earn all desirable outcomes—wealth, health, success, happiness, a good life.

The opposite holds true as well. By failing to exert control, by not working hard enough, people must bear responsibility for whatever outcome befalls them. If negative life events happen, it is because they are not trying hard enough.

The belief in personal control—along with an astonishing overestimation of what, in fact, we can control—has been documented in many ways. Some of the evidence is frivolous, yet quite telling. For example, people who buy lottery tickets prefer to pick their own numbers to those that are computer generated—yet the drawing is completely random.[4] Gamblers prefer to throw dice themselves rather than have the croupier do so—yet the dice still remain dice, no matter who tosses them.[5] Being in control of these chance events leads to a sense of heightened mastery, and a false notion that we can steer the outcome.

Similarly, to a degree that far exceeds an accurate appraisal of reality, we tend to see ourselves as invulnerable, protected, and able to avoid a range of catastrophic life events by exerting enough control.[6] We underestimate risk and overestimate a perception of our own invincibility. We allow that horrible things happen in the world. But not to us. They happen to other people—usually, we rationalize unconsciously, to those who deserve it or didn't try hard enough to avoid their misfortune.

We carry a semiconscious, purposeful disregard for the reality of all the terrible things that can befall us — illness, accident, violence, random tragedy. We know of these things. We read about them in the newspaper, watch them on television, hear of them from our neighbors. But we keep them far at bay. We try not to allow them to touch us. And when they do directly touch us—momentarily, piercingly, horrendously—we do what we can, wittingly or not, to brush them off so they don't stay with us.

Again, some consequences of this belief in control are quite minor. Does it matter, really, that I play my own lucky numbers when I buy a Megabucks ticket, that I imbue the numbers I pick with magical power? Probably not. But, as with justice, we apply this belief in control to social and moral functioning, with potentially dangerous or harmful impact. People tend to believe, for example, that those who live in poverty simply need to pull themselves up by their own bootstraps—that is, exert greater control over their lives—ignoring the complex web of political and social factors that create and maintain poverty.[7] Our underlying belief in control —a key to how we find meaning in life—shapes much social policy.

Along with these beliefs in justice and control, we also tend to assume that the world does not operate randomly, but by principles of cause and effect. Good and bad outcomes are not distributed by chance. If *x* happens, then *y* must follow; if I do *a*, then *b* will result. And these guidelines of cause and effect are determined by justice and control—the underlying moral principles on which we assume the universe is based.

It's not a far jump from these assumptions to an all-too-common tendency—"blaming the victim." We blame victims largely because of how negative life events threaten our implicit notions of justice, control, and cause and effect. If something bad happens, there must be a reason.

Blaming victims follows a perverse logic. If the universe *is* just and life *is* controllable, then when something bad happens, people must therefore deserve whatever negative things befall them. Victims must somehow merit their misfortune, or bring it on themselves. A woman raped? She must have been "asking for it"—flirting too much, dressing provocatively, consorting with unsavory men. She should have exerted more control. A gay man with HIV? He must deserve it—he is being punished for immorality, indulging in taboo pleasure. The presence of a "punishment" must imply a crime. There must be a reason, an "if *x*, then *y*" explanation. We blame victims —sometimes even when we are the victim—to reconfirm that we are right in how we see the world.[8]

When life goes smoothly, when the fit between what we unconsciously believe and what we experience is close enough, we don't examine our underlying beliefs in great detail. Our framework for life's meaning only rarely becomes the stuff of conscious scrutiny. It is like our heartbeat or our breathing: We do not typically concentrate on these activities, even though they are of course essential to life. We can become conscious of them, sometimes, simply by choosing to do so. But mostly we just take them for granted.

Yet when our breath or heartbeat becomes strained, we have no choice. The disruption demands our immediate attention. The same holds true for the unconscious pillars of our life's meaning. Ever-present and vital, we normally ignore their presence. We sometimes choose to focus on them, briefly and curiously, quick to ignore them again. It is only when they are strained that they demand our attention.

Small upsets to our belief system may require some tinkering here and there, but we strive to keep major overhauls to a minimum. We disregard minor discrepancies between how things are and how we assume they should be—perhaps by ignoring facts that don't fit, or believing contradictions will right themselves in the long run, or counting on luck to intervene as an occasional wild card. How useful our various defense mechanisms are in this regard—how deft our ability to rationalize, deny, minimize, or repress distortions between what we believe and what we see!

But what happens when something major hits, and our core beliefs are grossly contradicted? When the world, as we have come to know and expect it, is turned upside down? When the pillars of justice and control begin to crumble? In such situations, we face a profound crisis of meaning: How we previously made sense of the world is no longer valid or useful. And this is the central challenge of trauma—to reestablish life's meaning in a dramatically changed world.

People travel different paths to meet this end. Some attempt (successfully or not) to reinterpret the disrupting event as nontraumatic, thereby averting the need to alter their beliefs. Others admit the harsh reality of the trauma, and struggle (again, successfully or not) to find new beliefs that fit the changed reality.

Still other people hold onto their old beliefs with unyielding rigidity, at the cost of either their self-esteem or an accurate appraisal of reality. For example, a person may continue to believe that the world is just—but that he is being punished—rather than risk abandoning a belief in justice.

And still others plunge into meaninglessness. They find themselves unmoored, adrift, rudderless. The needed beacons of meaning that once gave light and guidance have failed them.

How can HIV affect an underlying belief in justice? We will hear a great deal more about Anthony, Lucas, and Francis in the chapters ahead. Each, in his own way, is coping well.

Anthony, after years of living with HIV, has abandoned a belief in justice. At first he felt embittered and punished, that his having HIV was unfair. (As soon as we start thinking about "fairness" and "unfairness," justice is invariably at play.) For Anthony, HIV violated an underlying law of justice—"What did I do to deserve this?" But he no longer feels this way. Now he thinks that life is not fair—*but neither is it unfair*. It simply is. Fairness, or justice, no longer registers as an appropriate yardstick for measuring morality or his own worthiness. For Anthony, in regard to justice, the world (and God) is neutral, dispassionate. HIV is neither reward nor punishment.

Lucas still believes that the world is just—but justice is more mysterious and elusive than it once seemed, and far less absolute. For him, HIV is clearly a gross injustice in the world, a deep challenge to his long-standing belief in God. He struggles to reconcile his faith with the stark reality of HIV. Yet he is unwilling to abandon completely his underlying belief in justice. Despite his "fights with God" about AIDS, he continues to believe that the universe is ultimately just, and it remains up to each person to strive to act morally.

Francis, conversely, saw his infection as a "wake-up call." In retrospect, he believes that he had been living wrong — too much sex, too much alcohol, too little spirituality. HIV has provided an opportunity to make amends. For Francis, an underlying belief in justice remains quite powerful. The world continues to work based on a moral cause-and-effect principle: He had been "bad," and now he is trying to be "good." By seeing his HIV infection as kind of a punishment-with-reprieve, Francis maintains intact the notion of cosmic justice.

Each of these men is attempting to meet the challenge of holding onto life's meaning in a changed reality. They follow different paths, but have all found a way to integrate their infection into a meaningful life narrative.

Of course, many people recognize the limitations of beliefs in justice, control, and nonrandomness, at least intellectually. But at a deeper level, these beliefs don't fade so easily. For most people, they never completely go away. How difficult to relinquish these most deeply cherished and ingrained notions of our culture, taught in childhood and reinforced throughout adulthood. The universe is just. Goodness earns reward and badness is punished. People get what they deserve. Those who fail aren't working hard enough. Life is not random.

And they don't go away, in part, for good reasons. First, they are not completely untrue. Exerting proper control in life certainly *can* improve our lot. Justice may or may not be stitched into the moral fiber of the universe—but even if it is not, why not strive to live justly? Acting from a sense of moral "rightness" (for better or worse) imbues many a life with meaning. And cause-and-effect principles of behavior may not be the only law, or the ultimate law, governing the outcome of life events—yet all of us experience their effect repeatedly in our lives.

Second, regardless of truthfulness, these beliefs can be quite useful— it helps to have them. Psychologist Shelley Taylor and others emphasize that the accurate appraisal of reality is not the best measure of mental health. Healthy, happy people *do not* accurately perceive the world around them: They systematically distort perceptions in their own favor. Sound psychological functioning is grounded in a self-serving misapprehension of life. Mental health is based less on seeing things as they really are than on selectively altering our vision to bolster self-esteem — what Taylor calls "positive illusions."[9]

From late infancy on, we develop a distorted, unconscious sense of ourselves as invulnerable, excluded from horrible cataclysm, and magically exempt from the commerce of pain that may jar others' lives. Such beliefs are of course illusory—yet they are desirable outcomes of *healthy* development. For although obviously false, these underlying beliefs help maintain a sense of well-being and productivity in life. When examined too closely (or frankly, at all) they are nonsense. But they may also be a crucial foundation allowing us to cope, and thrive, in what is in actuality a random and capricious world.

And third, we often cling onto our underlying beliefs out of the pressing need to believe something. People have a fundamental need to live in a world perceived as meaningful. The drive to order or comprehend our world may be a universal human truth. And so even when our underlying beliefs may be invalidated, we don't easily abandon them. They may even survive wanton challenges, such as those brought on by trauma. Despite the specific pains you or I may suffer, it may be a far *greater* disaster to risk losing how we make sense of the world.

In other words, the need for some framework of meaning is so pressing that it often supersedes the details or consistency of what is believed. An imprecise, imperfect, or even self-harming framework of meaning may be better than no framework at all.

Let's return to Daniel.

This young man had faced life events that could sorely test one's belief in a meaningful world. Yet he continued to meet the challenges in front of him with courage and optimism. In my meetings with him I was curious: How had he come to understand the dramatic life circumstances that had befallen him, particularly the untimely death of both his parents? As he spoke, it became clear that without consciously setting out to do so, Daniel had come to find some reason, some explanation, for their deaths. Yet interestingly, the meanings for each death were contradictory and arrived at through different paths.

Daniel was a devout Christian, and so was his mother. This was just one of several ways in which they had a close relationship; Daniel's sympathies and allegiance were strongly with his mother following his parents' divorce. When he talked about his mother's dying, he would smile, sadly but warmly. Wistfully, he said that "God took her for a reason, he was in control. . . . He knows what he's doing, and ultimately, he causes all things to work together for the good." Daniel took great solace in this belief. It comforted him to see his mother's death as part of a larger spiritual plan.

Daniel's father, however, was not Christian. Thinking about his death, he first said, "I can't figure out why it happened." He then went on, however, to connect his death with reasons quite different from those of his mother: "I think his cancer was a result of stress and negative feelings. I think he felt very guilty about how he left my mother and it was really eating at him, and that's what killed him, that's why he got cancer."

Daniel then added that he thought his father's death was somehow related to the fact that "he wasn't Christian." Yet this contradicted his assertion moments earlier that his mother's death was best understood *because* of her Christianity!

The two explanations of why his mother and father died were at odds with one another: Daniel saw his mother's death as reward, his father's as punishment or justice. It is as if his father somehow deserved to die and his mother earned the privilege.

Despite their contradiction, these beliefs are joined together at a deeper level. What unites them is the fact that some explanation, of any sort, is required.

I think Daniel needed to see some meaning or purpose in the horrible events that had shaped his life. He could not accept that they were just random or capricious. His thinking lacked logic, and made no sense when examined too closely. Yet so what! This seemed a small price to pay, given what might be, for him, a far greater cost: living in a meaningless world, where beloved people die willy-nilly, for no reason, with no fairness, beyond personal control, without being part of a larger purpose.

Meaning in the Worst of Times:
Lessons from War and Illness

Events of incomprehensible devastation and despair—holocaust, genocide, widespread disaster or atrocity—of course disturb us for the pain and loss involved. But we also fear them because of the gross violation they represent to our basic assumptions about life's meaning. As with HIV's crash entrance into gay life, such events have the potential to shatter the soothing illusory beliefs that help us get on with the willful, cheery blindness of ordinary living. From some of the bleakest pages of human experience, much has been written of relevance to life in the age of AIDS.

One particularly eloquent voice is that of psychiatrist Victor Frankl. A Holocaust survivor, Frankl founded *logotherapy*, a school of psychotherapy that regards the need to find meaning in life as the primary motivational force in human functioning. Frankl writes from his own experience as a prisoner in Nazi concentration camps. He survived the camps. His wife, parents, and brother did not.

Frankl's most influential book, *Man's Search for Meaning*[10] (which he originally entitled *From Death Camp to Existentialism*), relates his account of life amid the dehumanizing horrors of the concentration camps. The work stands as a moving testament to the courage that people reveal in extreme circumstances, even in the midst of the most heinous and morally destitute events.

Frankl describes a three-step psychological reaction to the horror of the Nazi camp experience. First is a period of shock. A new prisoner greets the situation with utter disbelief and a lack of comprehension: This cannot be. The shock arises not only from the horror of the situation, but also from its absolute discrepancy with all that has come before in "normal" life. Every aspect of a person's prior self-identity is suddenly irrelevant. The new prisoner enters a world that completely inverts the expected moral order of society: Compassion has been replaced by brutality, individuality by anonymity, interpersonal respect by denigration, a benevolent or benign environment by sadism, the natural safeguarding of life by random death.

After shock comes apathy. This becomes a primary psychological tool for survival, a "necessary protective shell"[11] that develops to protect a person from the inescapability of the despair, torture, and physical and psychological punishment of daily camp life.

This apathy, so necessary for survival, continues into the third phase, that of "post-liberation." Frankl vividly describes his experience, after years of imprisonment, of the first moments and days after liberation, for him and his fellow prisoners:

> We walked slowly along the road leading from the camp . . . we
> wanted to see the surroundings for the first time with the eyes of

free men. . . . We came to a meadow full of flowers. We saw and realized that they were there, but we had no feelings about them . . . we did not yet belong to this world.

In the evening when we all met again in our hut, one said secretly to the other, "Tell me, were you pleased today?"

And the other replied, feeling ashamed as he did not know that we all felt similarly, "Truthfully, no!" We had literally lost the ability to feel pleased and had to relearn it slowly.[12]

Yet central to Frankl's account is that, even as the horrors of the situation necessarily deadened a prisoner's emotional and psychological vitality, the very nature of the relentless adversity also provided an opportunity to struggle for meaning in life. For Frankl personally, finding meaning involved holding on to a belief in God and maintaining a sense of personal hope for the future. Even more crucial was a growing inner discovery of the transcendent importance of love—"the greatest secret that human poetry and human thought and belief have to impart."[13]

In his bleakest moments, and as a daily ritual, Frankl focused his imagination on his most cherished memories of his beloved wife. These private reveries transcended the despair of the moment. They also provided him with an inner armor stronger than any harm the Nazis could perpetrate against him. Torture, neglect, debasing humiliation: None of these could diminish the sanctity or power of his loving memories. Love was what mattered. It was eternal, it was supreme. The Nazis might kill him. They could not kill his experience of having loved.

Frankl argues that even in the most adverse situations, people retain the irrevocable freedom to make choices, to act morally and with dignity. To be, as he calls it, "worthy of their sufferings."[14]

He also observes that, despite the physical hardships and brutality of the camps, it was not necessarily the most physically fit who managed to survive:

In spite of all the enforced physical and mental primitiveness of the life in a concentration camp, it was possible for spiritual life to deepen. Sensitive people who were used to a rich intellectual life may have suffered much pain (they were often of a delicate constitution), but the damage to their inner selves was less. They were able to retreat from their terrible surroundings to a life of inner riches and spiritual freedom. Only in this way can one explain the apparent paradox that some prisoners of a less hardy make-up often seemed to survive camp life better than did those of a robust nature.[15]

The greatest psychological danger to prisoners was giving up hope. As long as a person held onto some faith in the future, he or she could maintain the strength needed to carry on. Without hope, the will to survive faded. When this psychological death happened, physical death was not far behind.

Other investigators have pointed out that concentration camp prisoners developed a range of coping strategies: a differential focus on the good; survival for some purpose; psychological removal, including intellectualization, humor, and a belief in immortality; a sense of mastery over some aspect of the situation; the will to live; hope; group affiliation; regressive behavior; "null coping," or passively adopting a fatalistic attitude; and "anticoping," or surrendering to the stress.[16]

The most effective copers relied on more than one strategy. In fact, overdependence on any one was maladaptive. For example, a person whose survival was guided by only one specific purpose, such as reunion with a beloved partner or family member, was at great risk for despair and hopelessness if he or she learned of the death of that person. Or a coping strategy based solely on group affiliation could be shattered with the breakup of the group, either through death or transfer to another camp. Prisoners who mainly relied on the last two strategies, "null coping" or "anticoping," fared more poorly than those whose coping involved some active components, mainly because of how they gave up all efforts at personal control.

Another prominent investigator into these dark corners of human experience is psychiatrist Robert Lifton, who has written extensively about surviving what he calls "massive death experiences."[17] Lifton has studied or interviewed survivors of several atrocities and natural disasters, including the Hiroshima bombings, Nazi concentration camps, a 1972 flood disaster that decimated a rural town in West Virginia, and American veterans of the Vietnam War.

Even across such varied events, Lifton notes that survivors of traumatic events exhibit common psychological responses. He highlights five themes that, taken together, constitute "the concept of the survivor."[18] Like

Frankl's firsthand account of the Holocaust, and the coping strategies of concentration camp prisoners, Lifton's "survivor themes" apply to AIDS and modern gay life.

First of these themes is a "death imprint." The death imprint is an indelible image of death that becomes lodged in the survivor's imagination, specific to the nature of the particular disaster.

Second is "survivor guilt." The heart of survivor guilt is the question, "Why did I survive while he, she, or they died?"[19] Survivor guilt stems from the randomness of the situation, the fact that survival or death may be largely a matter of caprice, fate, or luck.

Third, "psychic numbing" is the survivor's diminished capacity to feel. Like the apathy described by Frankl, this numbing may be adaptive in curtailing the emotional overload of traumatic events. But it can also lead to longer-term adverse effects such as withdrawal, depression, despair, and feeling dead or numb.

Fourth, survivors develop a "suspicion of counterfeit nurturance." They distrust the genuineness of help or concern that is offered to them. Their trust in a benign or benevolent world has been sorely tested. The reality of the traumatic event overrides any comfort that "things will be okay."

And fifth is the struggle for meaning. This arises because of how massive death experiences grossly contradict many of the rules by which survivors had previously guided their lives.

From his interviews with survivors of the Hiroshima bombings, Lifton also discusses the unique aspects of grief in events of massive death.[20] The Hiroshima survivors grieved not only for their most personal losses, but also for *all* the victims. They grieved for neighbors and acquaintances, for strangers, for the innumerable intangible losses of community and culture.

In any massive death situation, more than individual lives are lost. This rings true in our communities today, where dying has become a commonplace. Gay culture, as a whole, is engaged in an ongoing and continual process of bereavement. Ours is a world of grief.

Lifton speaks of Hiroshima and Vietnam—his images also describe Christopher Street and the Castro. War zones all. Frankl writes of life amid constant death; a visit to West Hollywood, or Montrose in Houston, or Dupont Circle in Washington, D.C., brings these words to grim life. Frankl yearns for transcendent meaning in a world clouded in despair. The essence of that struggle replays daily in thousands of our lives.

Survivor guilt may be more relevant to HIV-negative than HIV-positive men. A "death imprint" may be most pronounced in those with multiple losses (AIDS surely has a particular face of death, a specific visage repeated over and over, distressingly real and unforgettable to those who have seen it). Yet Lifton's survivor themes, as a whole, apply to us.

So, too, does Frankl's description of adaptation among concentration camp prisoners to their new lot. His progression from shock to apathy parallels the emotional trek of gay communities in the crisis—from shock to hope to rage to a weary, grief-benumbed exhaustion. We are not apathetic, precisely. We are burdened with an unending grief that depletes our energy. Frankl's supreme belief in human dignity, and his admonition to strive for hope and courage in even the most desolate of times, could not be more timely.

Like war, much of relevance to HIV has been written about the effects of living with other severe, life-threatening disease.

AIDS parallels both chronic and terminal illness. On the one hand, HIV has relinquished none of its lethal tenacity (although its deadliness is certainly less absolute than the media typically portrays).[21] Yet despite its high death rate, continual medical advances have steadily extended life *and* quality of life. People live longer without symptoms. Treatments have been developed for many specific ailments, both prophylactically and in response to specific infections. *Pneumocystis carinii* pneumonia, for example, had long been the leading cause of death for people with AIDS; now it is largely preventable and treatable, and its pervasive lethality has declined sharply. The phrase "living with AIDS" conveys more than empty optimism. It is an ever more sustainable medical reality.

What can be learned from other illnesses? Firsthand accounts of living with terminal, chronic, or severe illness abound, many of which are insightful and movingly written.[22] They capture the intensity and difficulty of the experience, as well as detailing the challenges to life's meaning that illness can so easily produce. As psychiatrist Arthur Kleinman succinctly notes, "Nothing so concentrates experience and clarifies the central conditions of living as serious illness."[23]

Perhaps one point, surprisingly, emerges from these many true-life accounts more than any other: Severe illness, even if terminal, need not be solely a horrible enterprise.

To the outsider looking in, the experience of severe illness seems completely dreadful, with no redeeming features. People sometimes wonder how an ill person can cope with or tolerate his or her situation at all. They make the assumption, "If *I* were in their shoes, I couldn't handle it."

Yet to the ill person, the situation is often more complex and ambiguous. Despite the undeniable hardships, there may be unforeseen gains: the strength that springs from learning that you can indeed cope; an increased awareness of the preciousness of life; the freeing ability to be more intimate with loved ones (how frequently people ignore the words "I love you" in daily life—how much easier they may flow when time is finite). Any or all of these gains may become part of how illness affects life's meaning.

Researchers have also observed this. In one study comparing HIV-positive gay men with noninfected gay men, those with the virus showed more signs of depression and anxiety than those without it. This is not surprising. Yet contrary to what most people might expect, the seropositive men also reported more life *enjoyment* than their noninfected counterparts.[24] The same has been documented in some studies of people with cancer: as a group, they report more life distress, *and* more life enjoyment, than healthy individuals.[25]

And so, for some people, the crisis of severe illness becomes a challenge for living life to its fullest. It does, indeed, "concentrate and clarify" some of the fundamental aspects of life. The fat is trimmed away. Life takes on an ever richer flavor, seasoned with the distilled essence of whatever matters most.

Another important aspect of illness is our pervasive tendency to metaphorize it.

Susan Sontag, in her books *Illness as Metaphor* and *AIDS and Its Metaphors*, examines the enormous power of metaphor on how we perceive, respond to, and treat those with illnesses.[26] She does not completely criticize the tendency to metaphorize or ascribe meaning to illness; to some extent, she sees the need to attach meaning to life events—including illness and death — as unavoidable. But the danger comes when illness-related metaphors are taken too literally, as fact rather than symbol.

When metaphor is applied rigidly, a person's unique characteristics are replaced by a one-size-fits-all fantasy about what he or she must be like as the carrier of a specific disease. The illness replaces the person. This is true with how we look at others, and how we may come to look at ourselves.

Throughout history, certain diseases have provided richer grist for metaphor than others. The bubonic plague in medieval times, tuberculosis in the nineteenth century, cancer through much of the twentieth century, and now AIDS. The metaphors of a particular illness are shaped by the era, the nature of the disease, whom it afflicts, and the social fabric of the culture at large.

Perhaps more than any other modern disease, AIDS is full of metaphorical meanings. It is sexually transmitted — and *homo*sexually transmitted — in a culture that not only abhors things homosexual, but frets about most anything sexual at all (our culture can aptly be described not just as homophobic but as "erotophobic," or fearful of sexuality and eroticism in all but the most circumscribed of expressions). AIDS' greatest impact has been among marginalized, oppressed, and disliked segments of society. It sprang, seemingly from nowhere, to mammoth proportion. It is lethal and mysterious.

And so to the culture at large, AIDS conjures up frightening, repellent images. The metaphors of AIDS are negative and damning. They speak of sexual licentiousness, sin, and deviant identity. They stem from our deeply ingrained assumption of cosmic justice: If you're being punished, then you must have been bad.

Because of these stigmatizing metaphors, life with HIV involving wading through the debris of public bigotry in order to reclaim a unique self-identity. These metaphors, borne from fear and judgment, rob people of their individuality. They render all with HIV the same. Everyone affected by HIV must tease apart meanings and metaphors that are self-created from those that are imposed.

Meaning, Homosexuality, Culture, and Stigma

Gay people are no strangers to questions of meaning. Long before HIV, most gay men and women have struggled with these issues of life's meaning, consciously or not, through the very process of accepting who we are.

Even in the most benign circumstances, coming to terms with being gay parallels aspects of a traumatized person's journey to reestablish the belief in a meaningful world. To be gay, we must reject, challenge, or redefine many of the deepest assumptions that permeate our society. Edmund White, who has chronicled the details of gay mens' lives (with and without HIV) in many evocative writings, speaks of this need for people to redefine meaning in the context of being gay:

> We could speak of that obligatory existentialism forced on people who must invent themselves. . . . Once one discovers one is gay one must choose everything, from how to walk, dress and talk to where to live, with whom, and on what terms. . . . The nature of gay life is that it is philosophical.[27]

Growing up gay differs from heterosexual development in some key ways. Starting as early as childhood, gay people are often forced into a stance of private shame and public pretense. For gay teens, many of the crucial tasks of adolescence go underground or even stop completely, given the absence of social and familial validation. All teens struggle with the new worlds of sexuality and intimacy, but heterosexual teens don't usually experience a fundamental aspect of the self—the core knowledge of whom one loves, or to whom one is attracted—as something secret, unwanted, or loathed.[28]

And rarely, unfortunately, are the circumstances benign. Even as our culture inches toward acceptance of homosexuality, the social fabric remains oppressively homophobic. Explicit condemnation or disapproval of homosexuality is common. Frank anti-gay hatred and violence are integral parts of the cultural landscape. Hostility, overt or subtle, may be routinely expressed in what would otherwise be the protected comfort of family. Growing up gay, for too many people, has the hallmarks of continual trauma.

As with other traumas, gay people have needed, individually and communally, to challenge norms to find meaning in life. Accepting being gay is a process of sifting through various ingrained cultural beliefs to determine what remains valuable, what must be discarded because it no longer fits. When successful, this struggle transforms feelings of shame, stigma, and self-blame into a greater sense of pride and self-worth.

But the process is not always successful. Many gay men and women find themselves unable to reject heterosexual society's condemnation. They view homosexuality as wrong or immoral, as punishment or sin. They may believe that if they tried hard enough, they would be straight. Such a stance often causes (and reflects) great damage to one's self-esteem. Yet, as with other traumas, this self-harming position may also, ironically, serve a hidden purpose—to maintain intact a framework of meaning.

Perhaps it is here that the cultural context in which we create life's meaning comes into sharpest focus. Meaning does not unfold in a vacuum. Public forces influence private beliefs to a far greater degree than we may think. Religion, media, family, government—these are our prime conveyors of meaning. To a large degree, it is through these channels that our basic beliefs are shaped and maintained.

For gay people, the homophobic backdrop against which we lead our lives is not just an abstraction. It has real consequences. Gay people are often denied access to traditional sources of social support, such as church and family. Our lives are typically denigrated, ignored, or caricatured in the media. Our relationships are not recognized by legal or religious sanction. The heterosexual widow who loses a mate receives a tacit level of social support and condolence; gay men who have been widowed may be more apt to encounter scorn, ostracism, fear, or blame. Coming out may mean jeopardizing the interpersonal bonds, and presumed social acceptance, that had been crucial to a prior sense of well-being.

These same influences are amplified when it comes to HIV. Coping with stigma, managing self-disclosure, deciding how much you feel comfortable identifying yourself with a marginalized group—all these challenges to life's meaning, relevant to homosexuality, are revisited. The process of accepting HIV is apt to reawaken aspects of coming out. Past accomplishments and defeats resurface. Being gay and being HIV-positive may begin to interweave—in terms of how to manage self-disclosure, openness, pride, and shame; in terms of needing to once again acclimate to a world where the previous rules no longer apply.

Meaning and Health

Are there health benefits to successfully reestablishing life's meaning in the context of HIV and AIDS, or any other threatening disease or trauma? This is an area of great promise in learning new ways to heal many types of illness, not just HIV.

The body is of course connected to the mind. Whether seen from the ancient canon of Eastern philosophies, or the Johnny-come-lately perspective of Western medicine, the essential truthfulness of a mind-body unity has garnered much evidence. Many things have been shown to influence wellness, sickness, and healing: hope, stress reduction, finding and taking appropriate action, even prayer. As the growing field of *psychoneuroimmunology* has demonstrated, how we think, act, cope, and express our feelings can benefit or harm immune functioning.[29]

Alas, it seems quite unlikely that we have within us a psychological "magic bullet" for defeating AIDS, needing simply to be readied, aimed, and fired. Yet this need not discourage. It also seems plausible that adaptive changes in emotional and psychological functioning can play a key role in fending off illness, exhaustion, hopelessness, or despair. There is much that remains unknown about the sophisticated interaction of mind and body. Some of what we do know is promising, and some of what we are now uncertain of may soon be taken for granted.

Yet there is an important flip side to discussing these issues, and a (loud) note of caution is warranted. More is at work here than the synthesis of mind and body. Equally relevant is our deep, illusory notion of personal control.

Most people embrace a mind-body connection in terms of maintaining intact their belief in the supremacy of control. We tend to see the meanings or course of an illness as generating from within ourselves, as if we can (and should) have the power to control it. "If I had been more attentive to my inner needs, I would not have gotten sick. . . ." "If I had been less fearful with expressing emotion, I would not have cancer. . . ." "I can visualize my invading enemies, and it is within my power to defeat them. . . ." If I am ill, I have not tried hard enough!

Again, the notion of personal control, so integral to how we make sense of the world, rears its head. Yes, much can be controlled. Careful and active stewardship of one's life has ample rewards, including possible health and immunological benefits. How seductive it is to get carried away with this—how easy to forget that the belief is also an illusion, an exaggeration.

What a fine line. To abandon control is often to give up hope; to embrace it too fervently socks the victim with blame yet again (often cloaked in deceptive words of self-empowerment). Despite its essential validity, placing too much emphasis on a mind-body connection—especially in terms of mind *over* body—is a doomed enterprise. The more we attempt to be in total control of our health, or our illness, or anything, the more we invite frustration and inevitable failure.

Still, the struggle for meaning remains a valuable, and perhaps necessary, enterprise. Regardless of how it may or may not affect immune functioning, living meaningfully affects the quality of life. This is something that may not be easily measured, but that can make all the difference in the world.

Summary

And so to recap: In each of our lives, creating and maintaining meaning is an ongoing, fluid process. Like our heartbeat or breathing, we rarely focus on it. Yet it is essential to the shape and tenor of our days.

We each create meaning in unique ways, while sharing liberally from the same pool of cultural beliefs. We tend to build this framework of meaning from a few central domains: by living for a purpose; by living morally; by effectively meeting our goals; and by enhancing our self-esteem. And to a degree that may be far greater than we realize, we unconsciously rely on certain illusions for how life and the universe operate: fairness, justice, personal control, and a moral cause-and-effect distribution of good and bad events.

Meaning usually lumbers along. It changes gradually, slowly, like a flowing stream whose course is determined by the accretion of subtle alterations. A cataclysmic downpour—such as may occur with HIV or AIDS—only occasionally redirects its path.

When an immense challenge does descend, however, we inescapably face the need to reestablish a new framework of meaning to fit the changed reality. People meet this challenge in various ways, with varying degrees of success. Some lose their grounding and plunge into despair. Others reinterpret the potential trauma as minor or nontraumatic. Others refuse to abandon their beliefs, even though they no longer fit, for fear of losing all threads of meaning. And still others transform the trauma into growth, through an arduous process of maintaining intact some old beliefs, discarding those that no longer apply, and modifying yet others to match their new circumstances.

As we will see in the chapters ahead, these basic responses translate loosely into four styles of adaptation to HIV: Rupture, Impassivity, Camouflage, and Transformation.

Not all cultures assume that the world is (or should be) just, or life controllable. These are hallmarks of Westernized societies. The need for meaning is universal, but the content of how that need is met is shaped by culture.

Eastern philosophies tend to emphasize instead the fundamental impermanence, unknowability, and uncontrollability of life. Justice and control may still matter, but only in a larger context of mystery and acceptance. At the heart of Buddhism, for example, is the notion that all things are impermanent and subject to change, including life, and that suffering is an undeniable aspect of existence.[30] How different this notion from the Judeo-Christian precept of cosmic justice, or from our twentieth-century American elevation of personal control to a supreme virtue!

AIDS is unprecedented, a new a chapter in the annals of medicine. It differs even from previous epidemics, especially when looking at the experience of gay men living with HIV. Never before has such a massive block of people, sharing a distinct but loosely defined communal bond, known with certainty that they harbor a virus of lethal potency and infectiousness —most often while remaining outwardly healthy.

And so AIDS' challenges to life's meaning are manifold. What an incredible brew, with ample ingredients each powerful enough *alone* to create a crisis of meaning. The recipe: grief (individual, collective, and everescalating); uncertainty (Will I become ill? When? With what infirmity?); stigma (Can I tell people? Whom? What will my family, my friends, my coworkers think?); mortality (How much time do I have?); and disillusionment (How can this be?). Stumbling across any of these individually is enough to threaten how to find meaning in life. Taken together, they create a crisis of meaning with few equivalents in the modern world.

AIDS has redefined our groundrules of love and pleasure. It has scuttled reasonable modern assumptions about health and longevity. It upends our prior expectations, hopes, and fantasies about life.

How have people responded to these great challenges?

3

Representations of HIV and AIDS: The Building Blocks of Meaning

Stan is a 48-year-old bank clerk. A quiet and shy man, he had never told anyone in his life that he was gay. Then he learned he was HIV-positive. Since finding out, he has done a complete turnabout, dispensing with his long-ingrained style of secrecy and guardedness. The results have been dramatic: At 48 and with crashing T-cells, he is just now, in his words, "coming alive." He describes learning that he was positive as the most transformative event of his adulthood.

At 27, Jules has known of his seropositivity for four years. These have been difficult years for him—a time of increasing isolation and loneliness, of anxiety and depression, of deepening separation from friends and family. He says, "I don't fit anywhere." He finds no sense of connection with his work colleagues, with other gay men, or even with other HIV-positive individuals. Jules has never lost a friend to AIDS and remains robustly healthy. Yet concerns about AIDS enshroud his life.

Eugene has adapted reasonably well to living with HIV. He has "good days and bad days," and suffers from bouts of depression. But he finds great meaning in his work with an AIDS service organization, and values the contribution he makes to the community. He has also found solace in rediscovering religious beliefs he had abandoned in his teens, 30 years earlier. His political views (another source of pride) tend to be progressive or radical—yet he also believes AIDS' presence among gay men hails from sexual "indulgence."

Stan, Jules, Eugene—each of these men's adaptation to HIV is shaped by the meanings he creates from his situation. HIV unlocks the courage Stan needs to come out, yet imprisons Jules in a lonely world of isolation. Eugene finds life more savory, even as he also carries the burden of feeling punished.

The particular meanings that each person brings to HIV determine how he is to live amid the brambles and thicket of the epidemic.

Our exploration of meaning and HIV continues by looking at specifics. What particular qualities or traits do gay men attribute to AIDS and HIV? What metaphors and images are conjured to paint the experience? What associations or connotations offer a glimmer of understanding?

I call these specific meanings "representations" of AIDS and HIV. Put simply, these representations are the ways gay men (and particularly seropositive gay men) see AIDS and HIV. They are how people have come to understand, make sense of, or mentally depict AIDS and HIV, in their own life or the world around them.

These representations may operate consciously. But they also may be out of awareness, becoming apparent only with scrutiny, by reading between the lines. Whichever the case, they exert a powerful influence on how people organize their inner experiences regarding HIV.

Among the men I interviewed, I repeatedly heard ten of these representations, spanning a wide range of emotions and ideas. I also found that most men relied on a small number—perhaps between two and four—as the basis to build their life's meaning. I suspect it is rare for a person's entire response to HIV to be based only on one representation, or to hold too many at once.

These ten representations are:

1. HIV as a catalyst for personal growth.
2. HIV as a catalyst for spiritual growth.
3. HIV as belonging.
4. HIV as relief.
5. HIV as strategy.
6. HIV as punishment.
7. HIV as contamination.
8. HIV as confirmation of powerlessness.

9. HIV as isolation.
10. HIV as irreparable loss.

Some of these are more adaptive than others. Some serve as valuable rallying points for a newly evolving sense of identity or worldview. Others are apt to be harmful or counterproductive. For now, my aim is not to evaluate their usefulness, but to describe them. For better or worse, these are the ideas that people turn to in response to the crisis of HIV. They are building blocks of meaning.[1]

HIV as Catalyst for Personal Growth

Many people discover that HIV can be a catalyst for growth. The potential trauma of AIDS becomes an impetus to move forward in life. A shift happens, subtle or pervasive, in facing the world. Things matter more. Life ceases to be a dress rehearsal.

Anthony,* who had a love of books dating back to childhood, enrolled in and completed a Master's degree in Library Sciences in his late thirties, all the while knowing he was HIV-positive. He found great meaning in his new work as a librarian. He also quipped, without much regret, "career gets to be a joke—I'm not looking to become the vice president or president of anything at this point."

Kyle, a 45-year-old man for whom HIV had been a tremendous catalyst for growth, described HIV as a "stern teacher" guiding him through difficult life lessons:

> I wonder if I would have the determination and the motivation to work as hard on my relationship as I do if I didn't know that I have this condition. That's the gift, that's the part I mean about the stern teacher. I think if I were not infected, it would have been very easy for me to play the game where life was about getting what I wanted, and getting comfortable, moving through and around people. . . . I'm not too sure I would have had the opportunity to understand what this life is all about. I don't think I'm there yet, but I have more of a view of it than I did.

Appendix A provides brief descriptions of each of the men whose stories will be interwoven throughout the book.

HIV-related growth takes various forms: Being more appreciative of loved ones. Reprioritizing values and time commitments. Discovering the beauty of nature. Becoming more forgiving and less self-centered with friends and family. Becoming more complete, integrated, or actualized individuals. Accomplishing goals, or partaking in activities, that would have otherwise been delayed or abandoned.

Some people find in HIV the impetus to leave an unfulfilling job or dissatisfying relationship. Some act on long-delayed daydreams of travel. Conversely, others decide to spend more time at home. Growth can mean pursuing a life dream that had long been shunted aside, or it can lead to giving up the continual pursuit of empty dreams and effectively limiting your scope.

Such personal growth is not unusual. Several studies suggest that most people living with HIV report at least some beneficial HIV-related growth.[2] Of course not all do, and people vary greatly in how central this is to their experience. Yet to some degree or other, this representation figures into the lives of many seropositive individuals. For some, it is a primary way of integrating HIV into a new framework for life's meaning.

HIV as Catalyst for Spiritual Growth

As a particular facet of personal growth, many people find meaning in HIV in spiritual terms.

Spirituality triggered by HIV takes several forms. For some, it is a nostalgic return to the church and beliefs of their childhood, or some modified version thereof. This may be accompanied by readopting rituals that had been forgotten or rejected. For others, who have maintained a religious affiliation throughout life, spirituality comes to assume greater priority. And in some cases, HIV leads to a dramatic reorientation of life to center on previously nonexistent spiritual beliefs.

Spirituality has been the central pathway for meaning for Lucas. Ordained as a Methodist minister in his twenties (prior to AIDS), he spent many years leading a predominantly heterosexual parish in suburban New York. He remained closeted as a gay man through those years, despite the frequent, unspoken presence of his "friend" Douglas at church functions. Lucas's decision to leave his congregation and focus instead on pastoral counseling with a gay and lesbian clientele sprang directly from his struggles to incorporate HIV infection in his life.

HIV has deepened Lucas's "spiritual journey." AIDS' devastation in the world, and his own infection, have been the greatest challenges to his faith that he has yet encountered:

> It's hard for me at times: I don't understand why, HIV now in my life. God and I have a lot of knock down, drag out fights about this one, because I can't see it. But there's a growing part of me that trusts God has a reason, there's something here for me. The questions of what it means are very much here with me everyday. . . . I've certainly learned an awful lot since I found out, and I feel like I'm seeing more.

He struggles — theologically, psychologically, personally — to reconcile his notion of a loving God with the horrors of HIV:

> God is sad I have it, but maybe it's more like God wants to see if there isn't a way to use it in some way that's redeeming, in me personally and in the world, in me as a microcosm of the world. It's in the Old Testament that "the devil meant it for evil, but God turned it into good." I believe that: evil exists, and AIDS is evil, but God can take evil things and turn them around into something good.

And ultimately, despite the challenges to his faith, he continues to frame his questioning in spiritual terms:

> I believe there's a force, which I call God, which is really the force of love. God is love, and I think that force is more powerful than any other force in the universe, and love can conquer and turn around any evil force, even HIV. I don't say that means that I'm not going to die; that's not it, we all die.

For Lucas, and many others, spirituality does not necessarily provide the answers for what HIV and AIDS might mean. But it provides the framework in which the questions are asked.

HIV as Belonging

Many men discover a deeper connection to other people through their struggle to accept HIV. They feel a greater sense of intimacy and kinship in their life. This is the third way people create meaning from AIDS: HIV as belonging.

Few psychological needs are more pressing or universal. The need to belong is central to society's major edifices: religion, government, nationalism, family, ethnic identification. It also occupies a central role in much psychological theory, forming the bedrock of entire schools of thought.[3]

Feeling that you belong to something, that you fit, can become a primary tool to find meaning in HIV or AIDS. Sharing private travails with others changes the perspective on our own plight. Believing that we are part of an entity greater than ourselves—a couple, a family, a community, a tribe, a social or political movement—can provide the sense of grounding that allows life's personal meanings to continue to unfold. How powerful the words, "I am not alone"!

Some people find this sense of connection with specific others—lovers, friends, family, perhaps a small circle of select companions. Leon, despite his deep sadness, also cherished the changes that HIV had initiated in his nine-year relationship with his partner:

> It's brought us closer together. It's forced us to dispense with some of the bullshit that we would get into, and try and really work out what's important in our relationship. . . . We'd been quite cruel and argumentative with each other in the past, and not respected and treasured each other for what we are, for what he is to me. Now, I'm very conscious of how wonderful some of the things are that we have.

Many men find this sense of belonging in a greater context: community. HIV can lead to a reinvigorated, or newly discovered, sense of group membership. The particulars vary—the community may be just gay men, or gay men and lesbians together, or a specific organization, or others living with HIV. The exact nature may be less important than the more fundamental sense of belonging to some larger group of people.

Many men have found that HIV can be a dramatic catalyst to strengthen their pride in being gay, privately and as part of something larger than themselves. They come to cherish their homosexuality with deeper fervor—a hard-earned reward for overcoming the stigma that permeates our culture. Kinship becomes a primary way to create meaning from a epidemic that has devastated gay communities and refuelled homophobia.

Craig's words capture the essence of this sentiment. When we spoke, I asked him if he had found any meaning in AIDS:

> No, it's senseless, it's just a disease. . . . What there *is* to be made sense of, and to be proud of, is the reaction to it, and to learn from that. On the whole, gay people have responded brilliantly: we've developed support works, support groups, groups to raise money and dispense caring to people who need it. We've learned how to deal with our own bereavement, on the whole, as a people, by insisting on acknowledgement for the loss, insisting on acknowledgement for the anger, and mostly for insisting on acknowledgement that it is happening, that these people are real people and not just statistics, not just numbers, not just fags, or drug users, or people of color that nobody really cares about anyway.

For Nate, being gay had long been a way of life—but, unlike Craig, one he accepted only begrudgingly. He'd never told his parents or four siblings he was gay. He dismissed all the "kissing and hugging in the HIV infected world—not deep kissing, but little schmooching here and there," as "too gay for me." He lamented that although being gay "had its rewards . . . they don't outweigh the penalties and problems."

Yet for Nate, too, HIV had resulted in a nascent sense of belonging and membership in the gay community:

> I think being positive has made me come to terms with being gay much more. I'm more at peace with it. I had never marched in a gay pride march before; I had gone to almost every one of them here in Boston, but I always stood on the sidelines with my bicycle, watching, cruising. Part of it was that for all the groups—and the Boston Gay Pride parade is a group of groups — there was never "my group" in there. I thought, 'Why isn't there ever a group that's mine?' Then, about two years ago, the question arose as to whether Positive Directions* should have a presence in the Gay Pride parade. I thought, if ever there were a group I should belong to in gay pride, this is it. So I marched for the first time. In fact, I carried the banner!

Positive Directions is a peer-led organization in Boston for people living with HIV. It provides support groups, educational workshops, and other social services to the HIV community.

A sense of community belonging may also overlap with religious affiliation. Such was the case for Eugene, who returned to the religion of his childhood, Catholicism, after a hiatus of more than 30 years:

> I've started to believe that there is a beauty in Christianity. It's something that I can carry, something that makes me feel warm, gives me courage, something that joins me with other people in a community of love.

And some men find in their HIV infection a feeling of universal belonging — a sense of participating in an universal community, beyond the confines of any particular subgroup or ethnic identity. Their connection moves beyond family and friends, beyond the HIV community and gay community, beyond the limited membership of their own particular religious sect. They derive from their own infection a sense of kinship with humanity, of inseparably belonging to a chain of humanity linked across the globe, through the ages.

With this aspect of HIV as belonging, the community is that of humanity, the kinship is to the people of the world. Eugene talked emotionally of the importance to him of a community of HIV-positive men. As he spoke, this sense of membership led seamlessly into a sense of greater belonging in a larger, less bounded group identity, transcending borders and differences:

> I wouldn't be able to survive without Body Positive [an HIV support organization]. It's empowering: the brotherhood, the camaraderie, the sharing, what we reinforce for one another. It's like people with any kind of cause, or struggle — there's a lot to be gained in the struggle itself, and sharing it. I get teary sometimes. There's this album by Dire Straits, and it has a song called "Brothers in Arms." I can get this sense of being in an army of sorts, of people that are trying to defeat a disease, and also the prejudice, and the discrimination and all the stuff that goes along with it. And hopefully, down the line there will be some sort of universal medicaid, universal insurance out of this, national health, and so there are a lot of things to be achieved.

For Howard, AIDS also triggered a sense of belonging in a universal community. But for him, it was grounded in the pain of loss, not the warmth of camaraderie:

It makes any awareness I have of how much people are suffering in the world all the more astonishing. There is so much pain going on, and my exposure to AIDS and people dying somehow makes all these people dying in places I know nothing about — it makes it more real. I can believe it.

A sense of belonging also underlies a central strategy that many people use to develop meaning in HIV: activism. For many men, political activity, or a heightened consciousness of issues about discrimination, offers both kinship and purpose — "What I do matters." Participating in a communally based movement for social change can provide a focus for feelings of anger, frustration, and disempowerment. How meaningful it can be to fight (quietly or rambunctiously) homophobia and discrimination; to rattle society's limited constraints about what is acceptable; to help create change that affects you, your compatriots, and others down the line.

HIV as Relief

In unanticipated ways, some men experience HIV infection as an agent of unexpected relief.

HIV comes, of course, with a long litany of dreaded features. Like any illness, however, it also has the capacity to liberate. In the process of coming to terms with HIV, some people find themselves freed up—freed from an overrestrictive fear of consequences, freed from the anxiety of tolerating life's uncertainties, freed from the weight of social censure. HIV may help some people loosen self-imposed pressures of "proper" behavior, or abandon stultifying social constraints. And, in particular, it can ease a burden of secrecy and become an impetus to come out after years of living in the closet.

Stan and Sam are two men for whom this was the case. Both were middle-aged men who had always kept their homosexuality well hidden, and structured their lives to maintain this secrecy. Neither had ever revealed his homosexuality to any family member or co-worker. Each had few, if any, gay contacts other than sexual partners. Stan's sole sexual and social outlet was the bathhouse he frequented until the mid 1980s; Sam typically met sex partners through personal ads. As a construction foreman, Sam joined in the homophobic banter and "fag jokes" at work to disguise himself.

For both these men, however, HIV was the catalyst to begin declaring their homosexuality in public realms of their lives. Once they did, they met with an unanticipated sense of liberation. For Stan especially, coming out after a lifetime of secrecy became one of the most significant events of his adulthood, a process that inseparably merged with being HIV-positive.

At 48, Stan had always lived a quiet, solitary life. He had worked as a bank clerk for the 25 years since graduating college. He had never had a romantic relationship, nor very many close friendships: "I lived a basic work, go home, and go to bed existence." When he learned he was HIV-positive in the late 1980s he assumed he would be dead "in six months." However, his bleak mood changed when he started attending a support group for HIV-positive men. It helped to hear others' stories. Perhaps more important, this was his first non-bathhouse social activity with other gay men.

Introverted by nature, Stan at first just sat at the meetings and listened. He felt too nervous to talk. However, empowered by the support of others in the group, after several months he began to speak up. To his surprise, he felt an unanticipated level of comfort with talking openly. So much so, in fact, that he soon decided to share his newfound comfort beyond the group's confines. After years of secrecy, Stan took the bold step of telling other people in his life about his sexuality and antibody status. I asked him what this felt like:

> It's like a great big sigh of relief. I'm never, ever going back in the closet. To no longer be isolated, to no longer have to live a lie, makes all the difference in the world! When I first found out [about being positive], I had no intention of telling anybody, and I lived with it for a year. Telling people makes all the difference in the world, like a ton of bricks off your shoulders.

Stan told his mother, his sister, his immediate supervisor at work, and then a handful of his co-workers. He became active in the leadership of an AIDS support organization. In fact, he had recently decided to take the courageous step of appearing as a panelist in a public forum on "AIDS in the Work Place"—a dramatic move at 48 for a man who had never uttered the words "I'm gay" to anyone else until he was 47!

Stan was quite eager to participate in the study I conducted. He began our interview by enthusiastically telling me, even before I posed any questions, "I have nothing to hide." After some polite chit-chat and a brief discussion of the interview process, I asked Stan to describe himself to me. He responded:

> I am a rapidly changing middle-aged gay man who is living with HIV. I don't really have any close relationships with anybody, and never have. HIV has really changed everything I think about and my whole outlook on life. Prior to this knowledge, I was not out to anybody, people probably knew but it was never discussed within the family. . . . Coming to terms with HIV has made a big difference. My life really goes around that now. I'm getting involved in different things, whereas before I was just a homebody.

I was impressed by Stan's ability to take such big risks after a lifetime of caution. His newfound ability to reveal himself publicly, and be more comfortable with other people, were steps of tremendous growth. However, his words reflected something even more particular than growth: relief. The changes he had experienced, beyond all else, were derived from the striking relief he felt, triggered by HIV: It's "like a ton of bricks off your shoulders."

HIV may also be an agent of relief in other ways, beyond coming out. At a deeper level of unconscious functioning, it offers relief to some people by lessening the ambiguity and difficulty of living.

Life is a struggle. We must constantly face new uncertainties and the anxiety of responsibility. Surviving, much less thriving, is rarely as effortless as we magically assume it should be. A fear of embracing life may shape our actions as much as the fear of facing death.

Writers as diverse as Sigmund Freud and Stephen J. Levine explore this aspect of unconscious functioning.[4] They argue that, in addition to life, the human psyche is also propelled, unconsciously, by a similar drive toward extinction. Seeking relief from the burdens of life may violate a conscious taboo regarding death, but it also may reflect deeply buried strata of the human psyche. Freud called it *eros* and *thanatos*, a life-instinct and a death-instinct. He came to focus on this topic more in his later writings, as his own mortality grew more prominent in his thoughts.

At a level that may be buried deep in the unconscious, some people experience HIV as potential relief from the perennial struggle of living.

The ambiguous is replaced with the certain, the unknown with the definite, the open-ended with the finite. Facing death can release you to face life. When the race is almost over, you can run with more gusto.

HIV as Strategy

In the early 1950s, sociologist Talcott Parsons elaborated the different social roles or scripts people learn to play, introducing the concept of the "sick role."[5] As Parsons explained, each of us knows, usually quite deftly, how to play a variety of roles in a range of situations—at work, home, in the community, and within our family.

The same applies to being sick. Although rarely made explicit, being sick follows certain guidelines and expectations. Sick people are supposed to conform to unstated norms of how to conduct themselves. There may be great tacit pressure to fit into the "sick role."

Some of these are akin to responsibilities. For example, we expect sick people to express at least some appreciation and gratitude to those who care for them, to acknowledge their newfound dependence. We also expect those who are sick to refrain from doing things that makes the illness worse —lest they lose our sympathy and support. (Note, again, the importance of "control." Our concern goes hand-in-hand with assuming that the illness is beyond the sphere of personal control.)

But being sick also comes with privileges. In particular, the sick are given leeway to act outside of standard social guidelines. An ill person enjoys exemptions from certain obligations and expectations, and has permission to receive a unique kind of attention. Rules that apply to others may not apply to them.

The same holds true with HIV. One way seropositive individuals may come to use or conceive of HIV is as a strategy to receive attention, love, or recognition. A person mines the benefits of the "sick role." HIV becomes a tool to wield, an interpersonal lever that can be maneuvered to fill psychological needs that would otherwise go unmet or undermet.

For example, HIV can become a strategy to receive parental attention. In Eugene's words:

> I told my mother and father [I was positive] about a year ago, because I wanted them to be a little more sensitive to my needs. . . . They weren't making enough time for me, and I used it in order to get them to make more time for me. I want to be babied a little.

They have four kids, and lots of brothers and sisters themselves, they're very family oriented, always running to this or that. So I felt, "Hey, wait a second—I've got problems, too."

And for Charles:

I'm careful not to use [being positive] as a tool to manipulate people with: It's easy to manipulate people by saying "I'm dying, it's the least you can do." Part of me wants to do that with my mother. I was going to take my mother and sister on a cruise. I worked very hard all last year to save up enough money to go and take them . . . my sister's going to go, but my mother canceled out. When she canceled, I wanted to grab the heavy artillery and say "I might be dying and may not get a chance to do this again."

HIV can also be a tool for public recognition, attention, or fame. Such was the case for Nate and Franklin, both quite publicly involved in AIDS organizations. Each valued the recognition he received as a result of being positive—a recognition they desired, but had not attained in other arenas of life. Nate talked explicitly about enjoying, and feeling proud of, the "urban celebrity status" he felt he'd earned.

For Franklin, HIV had led to some dramatic life changes. Franklin was a 31-year-old African-American man who had frequently lived on the streets and in shelters. He had quit drinking 18 months before we met, triggered by a "spiritual awakening" related to HIV. His sobriety was the key to start gaining a long neglected sense of self-respect. When we met, he worked for an AIDS organization, doing HIV-education outreach in inner city neighborhoods. In some ways, Franklin, the most troubled of the men I spoke with, had also gone through the greatest personal transformation. He described a sense of belonging, community, and pride that were completely new to him.

Using HIV as a strategy for recognition was also prominent in how Franklin created meaning out of his situation. Before getting sober, he said he used his infection as a strategy to earn sympathy from the many social workers in his life: "It was an ace up my sleeve." Now a public speaker in inner city communities about HIV issues, Franklin basked in the public nature of his new role: "I was on the radio a couple of weeks ago, and I enjoy doing that, I really do. I just love the attention, and that's being real."

Sam also relied on HIV as strategy to find meaning in his infection. As I mentioned, Sam had never come out as gay to anyone before HIV. At 50, he is now coming out with a vengeance. He has gone out of his way to tell everyone in his world that he is gay and HIV-positive: all his friends, his wife and teenaged children from an earlier marriage, his large extended family, even the entire lot of his homophobic co-workers. In addition to the relief he described at no longer living a secretive life, HIV has provided a way for this quiet man to suddenly enjoy the limelight:

The first few people I told were some cousins that were close to me, and my brothers. Just getting it out was really tough, to get the subject in that direction. But after telling a couple of times, I realized that it's a very dramatic moment, and I was finding myself enjoying the drama! I love watching the people's reactions.

Most people, I imagine enjoy dramatic movies: it's the drama of it, and observing people in a dramatic situation. I wonder if it's a little perverse, looking at it that way, but it doesn't *feel* perverse. . . .

[Regarding his co-workers]: I've had the urge to tell them for a while. . . Others try to keep it a secret from everybody, I have a tremendous urge to tell everybody. . . I couldn't tell everybody at once, so I started by telling my boss and his two assistants, at a time when all four of us could get together outside the office. I wanted their advice as to where to proceed: I wanted to tell everybody in the office, personally. Over the next month, I managed to get everybody in the office aside personally to tell them, some two, three, four at a time. I was willing to discuss anything.

HIV as Punishment

Seeing an illness as punishment is not unique to AIDS—it may be the oldest meaning attributed to illness. Susan Sontag observes that Hippocrates specifically dismissed the idea that God's wrath caused the bubonic plague, needing to do so because others viewed it as such.[6]

But AIDS is not just any illness. The theme "AIDS as punishment" pervades our society. For various reasons— internalized homophobia, an environment saturated in shame and prejudice, the need to maintain belief in a just, controllable, cause-and-effect world— many people with HIV see their infection, at least in part, as punishment. In fact, the notion of punishment is so powerful that a person cannot help brushing up against it in coming to terms with being positive. You may not subscribe to it, but it is almost assuredly there to react against.

Punishment is one of those topics that often lurks in the shadows but disappears when focused with direct light. Because of this, I did not ask about it explicitly in the interviews. Yet the theme of punishment came up frequently—most often in words intended to dismiss its impact. A number of men volunteered it as something they did not engage in. Roberto's spontaneous statement was typical in this regard:

> Sometimes, I can think "I was bad, I deserve this," but I don't really buy that. It enters my consciousness, "I was bad because I did this or that," or "I really deserve this because I wasn't careful in that situation," but then I think, that's ridiculous. No one deserves to get a disease, a disease doesn't have the wrath of God involved in it.

Yet while many of the men explicitly said they did not view HIV as punishment, its presence came through in other words they spoke. Most commonly, such sentiments were introduced with a phrase such as, "I don't think AIDS is punishment, but. . . ." These disclaimers seemed empty, given the words and thoughts that followed.

Whether explicit or not, whether publicly acknowledged or not, HIV as a form of punishment is a common unconscious representation for ascribing meaning to HIV and AIDS. A person may *intellectually* dismiss the notion of HIV as punishment, yet carry in his gut a disquieting belief that such unfair hardship could only result from retribution.

For the most part, this punishment is for a crime or sin quite specifically named: Prior to AIDS, gay men were too sexual, too hedonistic, too indulgent. HIV is a punishment for pleasure. Here are Eugene's words:

> We were playing with fire, and we got burned. That's not the same thing as the finger of God coming down and saying, "You sluts," but I was operating with the attitude "anything goes, there's nothing I won't do"—any numbers of people, glory holes, that sort of stuff, and now I look at it as being pretty disgusting. I'm getting back to my *Father Knows Best* sense. . . .

We went too far.... Back then I thought it was freedom, I thought it was wild and great, but my values have changed since I got HIV.... There was a lot of stuff to catch, a lot of parasites, and VD, and hepatitis, and human beings probably shouldn't have been running around, doing all that stuff and thinking that we were gods. We made ourselves superhuman in a sense, thinking that we were untouchable. Just do what we wanted, when we wanted, with whomever we wanted, pretending that it was all safe and nice.

Francis also comes to mind. For many years, Francis lived a rather lusty life. The pursuit of sexual gratification, in a wide array of forms, gave shape to his days. His goal in life was to find "the ultimate sexual experience"— and he had done quite a bit of hands-on field research toward this end.

HIV has led Francis to much personal growth; we will learn more about his story in Chapter 6. For now, however, one key facet of his response to HIV bears emphasis. How does he explain the presence of AIDS among gay men?

There was too much emphasis on pleasure.... For most gay men, pleasure was the only thing that was important. How they got it, where they got it, and with whom, didn't matter. It was the drugs, the booze, the parties.

Spirituality was a taboo word for the longest time.... Now there are a lot of gay men I know getting into all sorts of spiritualities, which they probably never would have done before. They're getting back to the roots that they should have kept, but they threw aside.

Both Francis and Eugene explicitly denied they saw HIV as punishment, but their words render their disavowals hollow. In fact, more than with any other representation, punishment is often disclaimed. Yet I suspect that this belief is quite prominent, or at least much more common than often discussed.

Although perhaps counterintuitive, believing in punishment may serve an important purpose: It helps preserve meaning. It upholds a framework of justice, of cause-and-effect outcomes in life. Believing that you are being punished risks damage to self-esteem—yet this may be a far smaller price to pay than seeing the world as meaninglessness or random. Again we return to a crucial point: People need to believe in a meaningful world. Sometimes an illogical or self-destructive framework of meaning may be better than no framework at all.

And so a delicate balancing act arises. How does a person balance maintaining meaning in life, but also preserve self-esteem? With illusion. Some strike this compromise by applying a belief in punishment generally but not personally—punishment relates to other gay men, other infected individuals, but not to me. The logic is faulty: If gay men are being punished, and I am a gay man, then it must be that I, too, am being punished. But the *illusion* of exclusion is helpful. Taking yourself out of the equation helps preserve self-esteem, perhaps until a time when you are ready to face the question of punishment head-on.

Others follow a different course, accepting the idea of punishment in their own life but dismissing it as a general theme for others. For Lucas, HIV meant revealing secret infidelities to Douglas, his lover of 15 years:

> I don't see HIV as a gay thing, I see it as a way of being gay that I messed up on. . . . I had a double life, and I think my HIV came from that: I would occasionally go to the baths when they were still in existence, and that was my problem, my fault. I didn't integrate that part of my sexuality enough into my life to not act out in that way, and I regret it.

Lucas waited two months before telling Douglas about his test result, needing to prepare for the possibility that Douglas would leave him. Douglas stayed: "It's been one of the places of grace in my life to have him be able to love me with that information." Douglas then went to be tested himself. For the fact that he tested negative, Lucas is "eternally grateful everyday."

HIV as Contamination

Related to punishment, HIV can lead to the sense of being tainted, pariah-like, a person marked by (or deserving of) stigma. This sense of contamination may be particularly acute in the early stages of being positive. For example, Nate spoke of the period of time shortly after his unexpected test result:

I remember walking streets and thinking that God, if these people knew I was positive they would stone me or shun me. That went on easily for a couple of weeks. . . .

When I first found out, I was going through problems with my boyfriend at the time. I was thinking that no matter what I had to do, I had to be thankful that he was paying sexual attention to me, because nobody else was ever going to do that again.

Nate intimated that these feelings of contamination were no longer relevant. Yet his words suggest otherwise:

In my relationship, it has kept me from wandering, kept me more on the straight and narrow than I'm personally inclined to be. I feel the pressure to be this way, because (1) I'm infected, and I wouldn't want to be out there infecting other people; and (2), it would be hard to replace my current relationship with something more satisfying—after all, I'm damaged and damaging goods.

"Damaged and damaging goods"—these words speak profoundly to HIV's impact on how Nate views himself and the world. Not only is he contaminated, but he is also keenly aware of his power to contaminate others. Harris feels similarly.

Everyone has sympathy for people with MS, people with cancer, people with any of a million other diseases. But to have a disease where the people are treated like pariahs. . . . I feel tainted, bad blood. I have a coat in my closet that has a little blood donor pin on it. For many, many years I couldn't give blood because I was asthmatic, but then there was quite a need for blood, so they lessened up on the restrictions a bit. That was such a wonderful feeling for me: I gave blood every six weeks, and I got a pin for giving so many gallons of blood. Now, I wear it on my coat for the irony: to have gone from a citizen of the state to a contaminated biohazard is ironic.

For Jules, a sense of contamination was not directly acknowledged, but instead projected onto others. He spoke about a brief romantic involvement with a man who had AIDS, and his need to stop dating him:

I know that my fear about having sex with him was very irrational. There was nothing really to be afraid of, because we were being very safe . . . but it felt like this person is dirty, or contaminated, which is a terrible feeling to have.

Charles was also painfully aware of feeling contaminated because of HIV. At the time of our interview, Charles was grieving deeply for a close friend, Tony, who had died the month before. Charles's grief seemed raw, palpable, undiluted with the necessary anodyne of denial. When I asked him at the end of our interview why he had chosen to participate in the study, he offered a spontaneous, heartfelt eulogy:

I did it for Tony. I think of how brave he was, and I draw strength from that. Realizing that every voice counts, my voice counts for something.

Unlike Jules, who could acknowledge his feelings of contamination only by projecting them onto others, Charles was all too aware of how he felt stigmatized. For him, HIV was both punishment and self-contamination:

It makes me feel tainted. All I can think of is what my brother would say: I'm a sinner. Also, I feel separated from people who aren't positive: It feels like there's a definite line between the two. . . . Being gay is sort of like the equivalent to having AIDS. . . . That's what most straight people assume as soon as you tell them that you're gay, that you're an AIDS carrier, that you're tainted and diseased.

I asked Charles what it was like for him to have contact with people with AIDS. As his answer led him back to talking about Tony, he began crying—both in sorrow and a fearful identification.

It's scary. There's still a part of me that says—well, maybe it's the way that people who test negative seem to feel about me. I know it's irrational, but there's a fear that I'm going to catch something from these people. I know better, but there's a kind of hysteria about it. It's irrational, but that's my gut reaction. It's hard to touch someone who has KS lesions all over them, or who is wasted away. Tony lost his eyesight. He was losing his mind. He started to suffer from dementia. He was seeing things, was in and out of reality a lot. It was hard to be with him.

At this point, Charles started to cry. Earlier in the interview, he had related to me another story that involved Tony, again one in which the identification—and the identification with contamination—felt strong:

Tony went to a party one time and somebody met him at the door and said, "You have AIDS, and we don't want you here." And these were gay people. So the discrimination feels real.

The knowledge of being not only infected, but also infectious, can be one of the most distressing aspects of living with HIV. Unconsciously, we all have fantasies of great, unlimited power, including the power to harm or destroy other people. HIV pries these fantasies out of the realm of unconscious symbolism and into the broad practicality of day-to-day living, particularly in matters of sex. Learning to manage HIV's lethality—as its target, or as its possible disseminator—can profoundly affect a person's sense of who he is, and how to create meaning in life.

HIV as Confirmation of Powerlessness

For some men, HIV fits into an already established pattern of how they see themselves in relation to the world: It confirms their powerlessness against larger, uncontrollable forces. For these men, HIV is neither a relinquishment of personal control, nor an affront to their sense of justice. Beliefs in personal control and justice have already been dashed by a sense that life is steered by the vagaries of fate.

Charles relied heavily on self-help groups to define himself. He identified himself to me as a recovering alcoholic, recovering drug addict, and recovering sex addict. With the help of AA, NA, and SLAA,* he had come to gain a valuable sense of self-acceptance that had long eluded him. He also attended many meetings each week. How did HIV fit into this? "I

---

* *Alcoholics Anonymous, Narcotics Anonymous, and Sex and Love Addicts Anonymous.*

don't dwell on it, it's just another part of life. It feels like just another meeting for me, one more disease to deal with."

Charles talked about being infected with the same resignation with which he has faced many life events:

> I was stomping around the bushes and had exposed myself to the virus so much that I feel responsible for my own infection. But I don't really blame myself: it seemed like one of those things that just happened, like so much of life just happens. I never planned to move to Philadelphia, it just happened. That's how I feel about HIV. It wasn't something I planned, it just happened.

Sam, the construction foreman, echoed these sentiments:

> I don't ask [why me?], it's never entered my mind. I don't know why I don't ask it. . . . One thing I probably picked up from my mother is a resignation to things that happen to you. If things happen, they happen—that's life. It's almost fatalistic. Anything bad that happens, I don't feel too badly about—if I'm poor, I'm poor. That's life. I can very easily adapt, take the attitude "C'est la vie" and not think anymore about it. If I'm lucky, fine, if I'm not lucky, fine, do the best I can—which I guess at this point is a pretty healthy attitude to have.

For Howard, feelings of powerlessness alternated with a rather strong belief in his own abilities. He perceived a very clear split between what he could and could not control in his world.

Professionally, Howard had distinguished himself. As an art historian, he had built an impressive academic career. He taught at a prestigious university, had won numerous awards for his work, and was esteemed as an expert. In this regard, he felt not only a sense of control, but a somewhat overweening pride.

However, beyond the limits of his professional identity, Howard's sense of control was greatly diminished. Howard is a black man who inhabits a white world. He has a white lover, white friends, white colleagues, white students. Detached from politics (both of race and sexual orientation), he is nonetheless acutely aware of, and enraged by, racism. Howard's previous lover, Seth, died in 1987. I asked what coping with Seth's death was like for him, and this led to one of the few moments in the interview where a characteristic emotional detachment erupted into tears and hostility—and the revelation of his expectation of powerlessness:

> Well, there's always been this feeling that life isn't easy, so it wasn't anything out of the ordinary. . . . It was draining, but being black is draining. The world never feels nice. People don't look at me like, "Have a nice day," it's more like: "Are you going to stab me or something?" This is a daily experience. Here I am: I'm professional, I'm 46, good income, whatever, and I can still walk into the grocery market and get shit on. So the pain of dealing with Seth didn't feel out of the ordinary. It didn't feel like life had suddenly dealt me a dirty hand: it was painful, but it didn't feel like it shouldn't be happening to me.

For men who think of HIV as confirmation of powerlessness, the question "Why me?" seems less pressing than it does for many other men. They expect life to offer random, capricious difficulties, even of great magnitude. Similarly, some men see AIDS as an ordinary, nontraumatic event—no worthier or different than other hardships, just one disease or horror among many, with nothing special to distinguish it. Anthony viewed HIV as a dramatic catalyst for growth, yet also found meaning and solace in reminding himself that "everybody dies, and a lot of people die horribly." Among the men with whom I spoke, Harris, in particular, seemed to try making sense of AIDS by seeing it as just one difficulty amid a wide array of adversities:

> There's not a disease out there that's very pleasant to have. AIDS is not the only horrifying disease. . . I don't think AIDS is the only problem our society has, either. Homelessness is a much bigger problem. And there's problems with abused children, abused wives, and all sorts of diseases that don't get enough research money.

HIV as Isolation

HIV can lead to a profound sense of separateness. Instead of forging stronger connections to others, it severs and destroys feelings of kinship. It can be an agent of isolation.

Some men experience HIV as leading both to greater belonging and greater isolation. Often, these are men who connect with other seropositive individuals, but feel ostracized within the larger gay community. Charles felt "separated from gay men who aren't positive: It feels like there's a definite line between the two." For Victor, who had felt like an outsider his entire life, other than finding a sense of kinship in New York's leather/Levi community in late 1970s, "even within the gay community I feel different, separated at times, because I'm positive, they're negative."

Lucas, the ex-parish minister, spoke of HIV as a dangerous wedge within the gay community. But in a poignant vignette, he also revealed how this sense of differentness had entered his own life:

> Yesterday, Hank, a very good friend of mine from college days, called. He had gone to get his test, and we had arranged that he would call as soon as he got his results. . . . He is negative. Needless to say, he was overjoyed, and I felt very happy for him, and very relieved. But after our talk, it triggered an enormous sense of sadness and loss. It took me right back to two years ago when I found out . . . I remember that feeling of what it would it be like to be negative . . . like having a near miss accident where you almost were killed in a car, and two seconds later you pulled away and kept going and were fine. I felt sad and angry that that's not the way it was for me, and very jealous of Hank. He asked me how I felt, and I said "Please understand that I'm ecstatic for you that you're negative, but the one thing I wish I could say to you is 'I know how you feel,' but I have to say, I don't know how you feel, because that wasn't the case for me."

The isolation of HIV may lead to an "us versus them" or "insider-outsider" mentality. It can feel as if only select others can know what you're going through, and that all others will mock or misunderstand it. The exact composition of the "us" varies: others with the virus, a handful of friends, a lover or best friend, a therapist. Perhaps nobody.

This representation seemed particularly relevant in the life of Jules, a sad, friendly, soft-spoken 27-year-old man. Jules had been living in Philadelphia for only a few months when we met. He had recently moved from Ann Arbor, Michigan, and had grown up and gone to college in Denver. Jules received his positive test result four years earlier, in Denver,

while still in college. He greeted the news with "absolute shock and disbelief." He was quite certain about how he became infected, and told me the
disturbing story:

> It was actually my first sexual experience. It was a date rape situation
> at a Halloween party I was at when I was 19. . . . It was a couple
> who had an annual Halloween party, and had a reputation for luring
> young guys who were just out of the closet into their bedroom at
> their parties, getting them drunk. I kind of knew that, so I think I
> set myself up for it, in a way. I wasn't prepared for how far they were
> going to take it. . . Between the two of them that night, they fucked
> me probably six or seven times, so if they were positive, there was a
> pretty good chance it was transmitted. That's . . . the only anal sex
> I've had without a condom, so I'm reasonably sure that's when I was
> infected.

The theme of isolation permeated most every aspect of Jules's life
history with HIV. After receiving the news at an anonymous test site, he
didn't visit a physician for over a year, partly because of his fears regarding
confidentiality in the university health system, partly because he could not
yet cope with knowing he was infected. He told nobody about being positive other than his lover. Eventually, Jules went to a physician recommended
by the Colorado AIDS Project. The doctor advised him to begin AZT, but
with no insurance, and AZT costing approximately $10,000 per year, "it
was out of the question." He didn't return to that physician, or any other.

Jules moved to Ann Arbor so that his lover, who was HIV-negative,
could attend graduate school there. Jules was unhappy about the move, but
his being positive played an important role in the decision:

> I felt that my goals and ambitions for the future were no longer as
> important as his because I was positive. He was kind of a control-
> ling person to begin with, and this gave him one more piece of
> leverage to put his own ambitions ahead of mine. It was a big point
> of contention where we were going to move, because I wanted to go
> to graduate school, too. . . . But he would explicitly say things like
> "My career has to take a bigger position than yours, because your
> future is less certain than mine." At that time, I felt like I couldn't
> argue with that. . . . I think I allowed myself to have less power in

the relationship because I figured, this is it for me, nobody else is going to want me if this relationship doesn't work out, so I'd better make it work.

Five months before I met with him, Jules broke up with his lover and moved to Philadelphia, a city he thought would be a good choice. He says that he is happy about leaving the relationship and making such a big move. However, his feelings of isolation and separateness remain strong:

> I don't think I have a very good attitude about my potential for having a relationship again. It's pretty hard to get a good relationship to begin with, and when you're positive, it's one more thing that makes it hard. I'm learning to focus on being happy by myself.
>
> I'm less open with people than I was before. I'm not very trusting, and I'm extra cautious. What it comes down to, I think, is a real fear of rejection that makes me feel less trusting: I don't want to let people know me.

Jules also feels isolated from the other HIV-positive men he had met. He occasionally attends an HIV-positive support group, but feels awkward about typically being the youngest man there (at least, in his perception). He has not been able to meet HIV-positive men his age. He also feels alienated from others with the virus because "I never led a promiscuous, wild" life. He returned to this theme frequently:

> There's the stereotype in the community that people who are positive were promiscuous, and there's a real judgmental attitude about that. It doesn't mean you deserve to be positive, but it also makes me angry because I never have been promiscuous, but I get that label anyway. It's a label that I find annoying, it makes me angry that the gay community is so judgmental to their own people.

I wondered, talking with Jules, how much of his sadness and loneliness related to HIV, and how much it might have been part of his life anyway. His isolation seemed to extend beyond AIDS—certainly, his detailed story of his rape seemed of importance in this regard, both in the fact of it and the quiet way he discussed it.

Listening to him, *I* felt outraged by what happened, and angry with the men who infected him. Yet he spoke noncommittally, with only a trace of resignation and sadness in his eyes. He shrugged aside my comments that the rape might still have an emotional impact on him, or contribute to his difficulty trusting people. He also dismissed several options I suggested for increasing his social networks, greeting each with a half-hearted "Yes, but. . . ."

Would life have been different for Jules had he not been infected at 19, or in such a disturbing way? The question, of course, is impossible to answer. Yet whatever additional factors complicate the picture, HIV has meant, primarily, that Jules perceives himself as alone. For Jules, to have HIV means to be powerless, contaminated, and isolated.

HIV as Irreparable Loss

Perhaps it is only in the ironic and bitter soil of loss that the seeds of personal growth can take root. Yet even when this growth is substantial, the cost remains inestimable. For many gay men—those who are infected and those who are not—AIDS is, above all, an agent of massive sorrow. What AIDS means is irreparable, incomprehensible loss.

It is both a dispassionate fact of science, and a terrible irony, that the crux of gay liberation—the ability to claim, and celebrate, our sexuality as a rightful and vibrant part of who we are—has led to this density of grief. Such is the nature of the epidemic that our individual and communal losses bleed together. Private losses resound at the communal level, and communal losses penetrate private grief. Like war, like natural catastrophe or human atrocity, our communities echo with loss. Boundaries blur between grief that is specific and general. How can you hear the pain of only one death when the sounds of dying reverberate all around you?

For Carl and Victor, HIV has led to a sorrow that envelops life. Awareness of loss eclipses their entire range of vision, like a dark cloud blotting out the sun. Here are Ron's words:

> Well, there are a lot of people who are dead, and it shouldn't be —it just shouldn't be. Now, everyone dies, but not everyone dies at 45 and 30. [Long pause.] It's the most serious disruption of my life that I have yet experienced. [Crying heavily.] It steals the time that was rightfully ours, and there's no replacing that. There were things I thought I had more time to do, relationships that I thought I had more time to savor. That whole process has been foreshortened.

And for Victor:

> I don't know if I really want to get old: There's not a lot of people
> left in my life, and I'm worn out trying to make new friends, have
> them get sick and die. I don't want to be old and alone, I don't know
> what value there is in surviving for the sake of just surviving. I
> think, most of the time lately, death might be a welcome relief from
> what this is, what life has become.... My life being visible and
> invisible have always been big issues, and every time somebody dies
> I become less visible. There's a lot of ghosts floating around.

One loss heralded by AIDS has been the demise of an era. An entire
way of life has faded. Remnants of the urban gay subculture that blossomed in the 1970s continue on, but they do so with the heart of celebration missing. Gay men's patterns of sexual and interpersonal expression
differ today from just a few years ago—maybe for the better, maybe worse,
but certainly different. For men who have witnessed the rapid disappear-
ance of a rich and multifaceted culture, this loss may ring heavy by itself.

The roster of AIDS-related losses includes the loss of gay cultural
norms, styles of sexual expression, diminished future possibilities, the premature relinquishing of personal hopes and fantasies. AIDS has infused
the sorrow of old age into individuals, and communities, that should still
be ablush with youthful vitality.

Yet amid all this, one type of loss clearly overpowers the others in emotional tenor: the deaths of beloved people. Grief over lost friends, partners,
ex-lovers, neighbors — this is at the root of AIDS' capacity to shatter
meaning. Coping with death after death, healing from one loss while
preparing for another, acclimating to youthful death as a normal occurrence—this immersion into loss has few equivalents in modern life. How
could such devastation make sense? How could this be?

Personal growth. Spiritual growth. Belonging. Relief. Strategy. Punishment. Contamination. Confirmation of powerlessness. Isolation. Irreparable loss. These ten representations span the diverse ways that gay men
attribute meaning to HIV and AIDS.

Of course, these representations vary greatly in some crucial ways.
Perhaps most obvious is how adaptive they are. Some are particularly

growth-oriented and hopeful; others speak more to despair or hopelessness. Some open new domains of self-exploration. Others constrain our ability to interact with the world.

These representations also vary in the extent to which we typically think of them as "meaning." In some ways, seeing HIV as an agent of irreparable loss or isolation more truly reflects an absence of meaning than the creation or discovery of it. These representations capture not meaning, but meaninglessness. They are "anti-meaning" responses. Yet I include them because they are basic to how gay men attempt to organize a psychological response to HIV and AIDS.

Perhaps most everyone affected by HIV can recall moments of glimpsing each of these themes—but usually it is a small number that shape a person's experience. The representations that occupy center stage may change and develop over time, with some rising into prominence and others fading out of view. They come together in varying combinations and with differing intensities. It is from how these representations combine that people weave a meaningful response to HIV.

And so two people may both see HIV as a catalyst for personal growth and increased belonging—but if one also believes he is being punished, this belief will color his experience. Similarly, two men may both see HIV as an agent of irreparable loss—yet how different their experience if one also sees HIV as a catalyst for spiritual growth and the other does not.

These representations can exist in any number of combinations. Opposite views often co-exist within the same person. An individual may experience HIV as belonging, yet still feel immense isolation. Another can discover in HIV both personal growth and irreparable loss. Human nature embodies contradiction; AIDS fits no tidy plan. In fact, acknowledging the paradox of these opposites may be a crucial step in living meaningfully with HIV.

Even though these themes mingle in myriad ways, typical patterns emerge. One cluster captures a growth-oriented response, and includes personal growth, spiritual growth, and belonging. A second cluster centers on despair and the destruction of meaning; it features isolation and irreparable loss. These clusters will form the basis of the first two styles of adaptation to HIV we will explore in the following chapters: Transformation and Rupture.

Part Two

Styles of Adaptation

4

Transformation: A Journey of Growth

Leon: This is it, you know, moment to moment, and trying to enjoy it, every moment. I'm not always successful, but I feel —not quite a pressure, but a strong sense that this is the only time we have, not next week, but now. Get everything you can out of living: do what you want to do, enjoy it. This feels like a positive thing, not a desperate thing—trying to treasure what's happening right now.

Anthony: One of the most positive experiences of my life recently has been my Body Positive group. Ten gay men who are HIV positive, two with AIDS, others with other problems, others just HIV and doing pretty well, and we all look very much forward to getting together. We have a camaraderie and bonding which is unique in my life, wonderful and really supportive. There's an easiness in that room, and a liking of each other, which is really loving.

Kyle: I know that I'm not getting away from this. It's real, it's here, inside, and how I choose to deal with it is key. . . . I've never had a very strong sense that I could get rid of this, heal myself that way, but I *do* have a strong sense that I can heal myself spiritually and emotionally.

Some men transform the somber, inescapable reality of HIV infection into a deeper capacity to appreciate life. They maintain a life-affirming

71

framework of meaning in the face of potential despair. They have learned to stay afloat in waters of great emotional turbulence.

Anthony and Kyle are two men whose lives reflect the style of adaptation to HIV I call Transformation. Let's spend some time here looking at their stories.

Anthony: "I feel utterly loved by the divine presence"

Anthony seemed an expert on issues of HIV. He was well informed, almost glib, about AIDS' impact—medically, psychologically, socially. He had ruminated over issues of life's meaning long before our interview. No matter what the topic—sex, death, religion—he spoke to me rapidly, animatedly, at times with a startling frankness. His manner seemed to be that of a quick intellect infused with, but not overpowered by, emotional vitality.

It's not a surprise that Anthony seemed an expert. He had been struggling with HIV for a long time. When we met, he had already known of his infection for nine years. In December 1981, Anthony responded to a researcher's ad in the *New York Native* seeking gay men with persistently swollen lymph glands. This was in the early days of the epidemic—before the term "AIDS," before the discovery of HIV, just months after the first mysterious cases of unexplained illness and death among gay men.[1] Whatever was causing these deaths, Anthony fit the description: He had generalized lymphadenopathy and his T-cells were abnormal. He knew he was infected and at risk.

Anthony had just moved to Manhattan two months earlier. He left his native Philadelphia because he was tired of frequent weekend commutes to enjoy New York's "party scene." He was 30 years old, had been out for years, and loved being gay—the discos, the baths, the sex, the drugs, the alcohol. Coming of age in the exuberant gay subculture of the 1970s opened his eyes to a whole new world. It gave his life a diversity and enrichment that far exceeded the boundaries of his working class, Italian, South Philly ("*Rocky* country") upbringing:

> I came out into gay liberation and I came out kind of noisily and
> politically and raucously. . . . In a lot of ways, my gayness, and early
> recognition of it, has isolated me and made me feel different, and

that differentness is fundamental to who I am . . . but the gayness has also pushed me. . . . Being gay has gotten me to meet people who I never would have met. My life, as a gay person, extends into so many more realms than I think it would have had I been straight, because in so many gay activities you meet people from so many different walks of life, since the only reason we're together is gayness. . . . That is what is most exciting about being gay.

After coming out in his twenties, Anthony immersed himself in the burgeoning post-Stonewall gay subculture. He moved to the heart of Philadelphia's gay district. He took only bartending and waiting jobs, so that work would not interfere with the rituals and pleasures of nightlife. His political activities dwindled as his passion for partying grew. Life "revolved around discos, and the drugs, the sex, the dancing."

Yet Anthony also felt restless. He was quite bright, with many intellectual and literary interests. In fact, he was the only member of his family to attend and graduate college—a "differentness" from them perhaps as significant as his sexuality. So at 30, moving to New York for the lavish gay life was also, in part, to beg off a disturbing, nagging question: "The other side of this was I was a person of promise and intellect. Why was I simply doing Quaaludes and working as a waiter?"

At that time, Anthony's response to feeling dissatisfied with his life was to throw himself deeper into partying. And then in 1981 he participated in that early AIDS study. Amid the terrible awareness of steadily mounting gay deaths, frightened by the knowledge of his own risk, everything started to unravel. When he learned that he was ill, or potentially ill, or may become ill at any moment, he responded by—partying more.

In the early 1980s, despite knowing he was infected with whatever it was, Anthony clung to the same lifestyle he had relished in earlier years. But it no longer brought joy; partying became darker, and far less pleasurable. Even the casual and anonymous sexuality of his past now felt too "intimate." He stopped going to discos—too much friendly chatter—and hung out at the Mineshaft instead.* He stopped tricking at home or the baths,

---

*The Mineshaft was a well-known watering hole for gay men on the outskirts of Greenwich Village, a bar whose popularity stemmed from the casual, and rather uninhibited, sex that was available. It closed in 1985.

no longer wanting to engage in the minimal polite, banal banter that accompanied these sexual trysts. He preferred the "darkness and efficiency" of backrooms "so I wouldn't have to talk." On a nightly basis he would go out, get drunk, and purposely engage in unsafe sex.

> At first, it was about me trying to kill myself. I wanted to die, so I did things like rim somebody, or blow somebody, doing things that would infect me. . . . The sex was about being furtive, I didn't want people to know me. That was the chief thing: not to have anybody know me . . . I felt like a wimp for using a rubber, so I never fucked [as a top]. And I would never think of asking someone in a casual sex joint to put one on, even though I knew I was supposed to . . . I thought I'd get to know them first and tell them, and that would be more forthright, but that never happened. . . . I even would let people blow me, and I'd come in their mouths. I remember saying to a shrink later on, "It's their lives, if they're stupid enough to have someone come in their mouths, that's their problem."

Anthony kept this going for several more years. What ultimately served as the key to turning his life around was getting his drinking under control. He began attending gay AA meetings. He was dubious at first, but willing to give it a try. He was not sure he was an alcoholic, but he knew he hated his life. The exuberance that brought him to New York had long since festered into bitterness, despair, rage, and constant thoughts of suicide.

Even without HIV, Anthony's life story may have been one of the healing power of AA to change a path of self-destructiveness. But Anthony *was* HIV infected, and for him gaining sobriety could not be disentangled from his struggle to accept the reality of his infection. Anthony's alcohol and drug use had become his primary defensive weapon against the pains of his life—and the pain that was greatest, and most unbearable, was HIV.

Slowly, getting sober allowed Anthony to steer his life in a new direction. The glitter of gay party life had been quite seductive earlier, even though he stayed with it long after the allure had faded. Now he wanted more challenge. In 1986, he decided to return to school. He enrolled in a Master's program in Library Sciences. This was, of course, by now well into the epidemic, and almost five years since he knew of his infection; his HIV status was confirmed by an antibody test the year before.

Anthony earned his Master's degree, specializing in rare books and old religious manuscripts. He got a job at a university library. In his late thirties, seven years into knowing he was seropositive, he began to savor, for the first time, getting up in the morning to go to work.

At the same time, Anthony also came to place increased importance on spirituality. This included "consciously relying on AA and its philosophy to guide my life." It also took the form of re-embracing his Roman Catholic upbringing.

A few religious themes were particularly important for Anthony in creating a sense of meaning out of his life in the context of HIV and AIDS. Among these were the idea of accepting suffering, and believing in the resurrection of Christ:

> You'd think that facing a fatal disease, facing death, facing all these things that in twentieth century consumerist, capitalist, happy-go-lucky America we're not supposed to face at my age, you'd get smart in some ways. I think the fantasy is that lying on the death bed you're going to have a knowledge that others don't have: well I do. I have a knowledge of suffering and redemption. . . . In some ways, I feel like I have nothing interesting to say about the meaning of life, about how to face the world, about my place in the world because of AIDS. . . . But in other ways, I could say to somebody, "I have compassion." I could say to somebody who's suffering, "I'm suffering too, and I know what suffering is about, and there are ways of facing suffering and keeping on going."
>
> I want to grow along spiritual lines, and part of my spiritual path is dealing with AIDS. I have to think that this is my suffering, it's been given to me, what am I going to do with it? I think of Jesus on the cross screaming, "I don't want to be here," and I scream, "I don't want to be here," and then I think of Jesus saying, "I accept being here," and I think—"Well, I'll get there."
>
> . . . This is the first time I've ever said this to another person, but I believe in the resurrection. Jesus died, he came back three days later. I don't know how he came back, I don't know what that was about, but I know he came back. I certainly, absolutely believe that, even though I don't understand it—well, yes, I do. In AA, I see resurrection all the time. I see people coming back to life . . . now don't quiz me too much on how I think after I'm dead, Anthony is

going to continue in a resurrected form. I don't know how, but I think I will.

Anthony's spiritual awakening did not lead him to rejoin any church or congregation. He didn't participate in any AIDS-related political activity, because he lacked "the emotional wherewithal" to put up with it:

In New York, the political scene is kind of pushy and demanding. And that's what it's about, it should be pushy and demanding . . . but I feel like I don't have the energy for it and it's not me.

However, he did find a great sense of gay community connectedness through his AA participation, and his involvement with Body Positive, an HIV support group. He felt deeply proud of the gay community's response to AIDS. He saw learning to accept HIV in his life as a maturation process mirrored in the larger gay community: moving from partying to seriousness, from frivolity to depth.

Through the trial and the adversity I think we [the gay community] are going to get stronger. . . . I've made sense of AIDS for myself in that a lot of people die, and people die horribly. I may have thought that my life was going to be one party after another, and that's not happening. It's up to me to accept what's happening in my life or not.

When we spoke, Anthony's psychological journey with HIV had followed the perilous twists and turns of many years. He had seen an enormous number of friends and acquaintances die. He had been on AZT for years, as well as various other experimental treatments. He was healthy, but had a T-cell count of 57. Despite the longevity of his growth and survival, he entertained no fantasy that he would be luckily or magically spared—he saw his likelihood of developing AIDS as "absolutely 100%."

As I later reflected on Anthony's interview, I came to think that his musings about resurrection gave him words, for the first time, to articulate his subconscious understanding of his own life narrative. Resurrection was the key: He had lived it. Thinking about his story, his life *had* been one of resurrection: through gaining sobriety, through returning to school, through accepting the "suffering" of HIV and AIDS and growing because of it. At one point as we spoke, Anthony interrupted himself. He paused for a moment, smiled a private, inner smile, and said:

> I don't know if it's because of thinking about death that I think this, but I feel utterly loved by the divine presence, however you want to characterize it—the divine mother, god, whatever.

He smiled again, like a bookend on the other end of that thought, and returned to the same brisk, frank style that characterized the rest of the interview.

Kyle: "HIV has been this stern, stern teacher"

When Kyle and I met, he was in his third year of employment at an AIDS service organization. A charismatic and handsome 45-year-old man, Kyle exuded not only charm, but a sense of robust health and vitality. His eyes sparkled. He struck me as one of those people who was either lucky genetically, or had learned some coveted, mysterious secret that eludes most of us: He radiated vigor. Long after our meeting, the glow of his presence lingered in my memory, even as the details of his words and looks faded.

Kyle had known he was HIV-positive for five years. He found out at the same that his lover, Frank, was diagnosed with AIDS. The news "astounded" both of them: This was 1984, and the two had been living a quiet rural life, far away from mainstream gay society. They assumed AIDS was a city thing; they thought they had nothing to worry about.

So although Frank had experienced continual weight loss and various illnesses for at least two years, the two did not believe—or refused to acknowledge—that Frank's difficulties were HIV-related. They had unsuccessfully attempted to treat Frank's ever-worsening health with homeopathy. Despite all efforts, Frank remained in great pain and was obviously ill. He finally went to a mainstream physician, who diagnosed him with PCP. He was immediately hospitalized, and died days later.

This had been Kyle's first gay relationship since he was a teenager. Kyle got married at the age of 22. At the time, he told his wife about his attractions to men, but promised not to act on them. He kept his promise, but divorced her 11 years later, impelled by the need to explore and rediscover the homosexuality he had long been suppressing.

Looking back on his life, Kyle always knew he was gay—or rather, he grew up "floating in the medium" of loving other boys and men, without the constraints and complications of a label for these feelings:

> My childhood memories are marvelous, outside sex and casual sex as a boy. . . . It was a world in which the concept of being gay hadn't been articulated yet, so it was much easier for us just to act and not have a label on it. Nobody was really watching or judging, there was no issue about it. I loved that. I look back on it as a state of grace.

Kyle met Frank shortly after his divorce. They settled into a domestic, easygoing life, not dissimilar to his marriage. Kyle, who held a Master's degree in English Literature and had taught high school, took up landscaping and gardening. Each had occasional sexual liaisons outside of the relationship. These anonymous encounters were tacitly acknowledged, but not discussed. Neither thought them a major problem.

The time immediately following the double trauma of Frank's death and the knowledge of his own infection was, by far, "the most difficult period" of Kyle's life. For six months, he experienced aimless grief, isolation, and despair: "That was a pretty bleak time . . . I saw this as a disaster rather than as an opportunity to learn more." However, his despair began lifting after this period of intense grief. He recalls one day realizing, "I'm probably not going to be dying anytime soon. I've got time here. What am I going to do with this time?"

An important turning point came a year or so after Frank's death. Kyle had applied to visit a spiritual retreat center he had frequented over the years. Despite his previous welcome, the center turned down his request to visit. He was denied because of his HIV status. His anger at this discrimination rallied and focused his energy: He became intent on changing the policy of the spiritual center regarding HIV, not necessarily for himself but for others down the line.

For the first time since Frank's death, Kyle had "a mission"—to change the center's policy. He had felt a sense of mission in his life before, but never one he thought as important, or as communally based. In retrospect, he saw how such previous "missions" had been for his own gain only. Now, he was beginning to identify as a member of a group. He was a gay man, a gay man with HIV.

Kyle also decided to move to Manhattan. For the first time in his life, at the age of 40, he became part of an urban gay community. He had always before stayed "on the periphery" of gay life. His exclusion from the spiritual retreat center, and his increasing involvement in gay life, opened his eyes to issues of discrimination and oppression that he had never before registered as meaningful:

> I've lived as a very privileged person, a well-educated, upper middle-class white male. In this society, I can swim in any water I want to swim in, and I thought all people have that choice. That's the myth this culture wanted to hand me. Once I really got a whiff of how disenfranchised gay people are, and how hard it is to be gay, it became an increasingly irrevocable choice for me that I want to identify as a gay man. I *want* people to know I'm gay. I want to be part of my era as a gay man.

Kyle considered returning to teaching, but instead pursued HIV-related work. He took a job with an AIDS service organization, where he eventually found his niche facilitating groups for men who had just tested positive. This work became the hub of his life, and the foundation of his newly emerging identity as a gay man and member of the gay community.

Kyle's work began to have a transformative, curative effect on his grief over Frank and his own infection. At one level, he did his job well, and freely admitted the importance of receiving others' recognition, commendation, and praise. But, more important, helping others cope with their infection provided the key to creating meaning in his life. His work took on an importance far beyond the details of the job. He laughed when he described himself to me as "a woman with a mission":

> Early on, I saw myself as an instrument: I've survived, there's something that I can help other people with here. This is my way of integrating what's happened to me, as well as integrating myself into a larger community. . . . At my most arrogant, in these groups that I lead, it's almost like I'm an initiator, or an elder for these men who have just learned they're positive. It's a wonderful feeling and I watch myself carefully so I don't abuse it, but I think, this is a rite of passage and I'm their initiator in a way. I'm one of the first

people they see who's made some personal meaning out of being HIV-positive, and that's my wish for them, that they make their own meaning out of it. . . . In the work that I do, I feel a sense of real connectedness with those men.

Another important development happened when he moved to New York: He met a new lover, Pete. They had been together for almost four years when we spoke. Pete, who is HIV-negative, has been an invaluable support: "I've healed more through him than anything else, and that's what encourages me to go on." Still, Kyle's infection was, and remains, a constant presence in their lives:

> One part of me was expecting that with this new relationship with Pete, I could deny that all this happened with Frank. I felt I could start my life over again, with the benefit of knowing that life was very precious and it did have an end. I'd had a stern mortal warning, and I was ready to work harder at a relationship, and harder at being conscious of my life in general. But I soon realized HIV was not going to go away. It wasn't something I was going to be able to outrun or deny. We're always incorporating it into our lives.

For Kyle, HIV has sparked a sense of tremendous growth and new meaning in his life. He personified his HIV infection as his "teacher":

> HIV has been this stern, stern teacher, the only force in my life that I couldn't charm away, I couldn't slither around. It's been a teacher in the very best sense of the word, and its only through AIDS that I've come to understand what the true role of a teacher is: it's not to be a friend, or a comforter, it's to be a guide, to see something there that needs to be brought out, sparked, in conflict.

Kyle has come to see life as a spiritual quest leading to deepening love and understanding. It is a mindset that sometimes eludes him—he puts great stock in the "creative denial" he uses to distance himself from the never faraway possibility of lapsing back into his sense of despair. But he has nonetheless created a valuable network of inner beliefs to impart meaning to his life. He has integrated the reality of HIV into a framework of meaning that allows him not only to survive, but to thrive.

Against the bleak backdrop of AIDS—or, paradoxically, because of it —many HIV-positive individuals have forged beneficial, rewarding, and, in some cases, life-transforming meaning out of their situation. Faced with the unalterable fact of their HIV infection, men such as Kyle and Anthony have transformed despair into challenge, psychological disequilibrium into a catalyst for growth, a "death sentence" into a reinvigorated zest for life.

Transformation is the first of four styles of overall adaptation to HIV that we will explore. By *adaptation*, I mean something broader than coping, broader than particular strategies to manage stress, broader than the specific HIV representations that form the foundations of meaning. All of these are components of adaptation. These four styles of adaptation paint the bigger picture—a more encompassing view of people's total emotional, behavioral, and cognitive response to great adversity.

It's important to note that any view such as this risks, by necessity, missing the trees to survey the forest. These are general patterns, not exact blueprints. Noe are they fixed entities—meaning-making is a constantly evolving endeavor. My aim with these four styles is to describe the ways I have seen gay men integrate HIV and AIDS into their life's meaning.

Nor do these styles translate neatly into current categories of psychiatric diagnosis. Still, there is some overlap. Men who fit the style of Rupture, for example, may be most likely to suffer from major depression or post-traumatic stress disorder. Some of the men who have a style of Impassivity rely on avoidance as a characteristic means of coping. Those who fit the description of Camouflage may have different characterological difficulties. But depression or anxiety can be present in all the styles, as can various traits of what are currently classified as "personality disorders." How a person meets extreme adversity is not necessarily the same as how he or she functions in more benign circumstances.

And Transformation is a good place to begin. The fact that HIV can spark growth, or even lead to profound life change, should not really surprise us. As a culture we tend to believe, superstitiously, that growth and loss must be kept completely separate—the two cannot commingle. We often carry a deep sense of discomfort, or even taboo, acknowledging that adversity or trauma can have benefits: to do so often seems awkward, disrespectful, even foolish. After all, how can you derive gain from something horrible—doesn't that diminish the horror? It is as if by finding any positive aspect of a trauma, any growth from loss, any boon from a bane, we sully our claim to rightful hardship.

Yet this too harsh separation of growth and loss belies many people's experience. The two can commingle, and often do. Growth and loss are better thought of as a continuum than as distinct entities. Every major growth contains aspects of loss. Even the most wrenching loss contains the seeds of potential growth.

Bereavement offers a good example. Surviving the death of a loved one is certainly an event of profound loss, a potentially devastating emotional experience. Yet some people emerge from their grieving process with unexpected gains. By weathering emotional tribulations they had thought unendurable, they have a deeper, surer sense of their strength. By facing despair and not succumbing, they know their own inner capacities in a more complete way. These gains do not in any way diminish the fact of the loss. But yes, they are benefits. Dearly purchased, hard-earned benefits.

So it is with HIV and AIDS. These are profound adversities. And some people respond to such massive upheaval not only with resilience, but with a remarkable capacity for growth.

In *Surviving AIDS*, Michael Callen described his own journey of living with AIDS, as well as those of other "long-term survivors" (now commonly refered to as long-term non-progressors). Callen was, among other things, a pioneering AIDS activist. He was first diagnosed with an HIV-related infection in 1982, and remained a vital force in the AIDS political world until his death in 1993.

For Callen, AIDS led to a tremendous sense of revitalization and personal growth. He likened AIDS to "a cosmic kick in the ass—a challenge to *finally* start living":

> While I would never have wished for AIDS, the plain truth is that I'm happier now than I've ever been. . . . AIDS has taught me the preciousness of life and the healing power of love. I've been more productive than at any time prior. . . . I've tried to see AIDS as a challenge to begin living, instead of a sign to begin dying. AIDS forced me to take responsibility for my own life—for the choices I had made and the choices I could still make. For better or worse, AIDS has made me the man I am today.[2]

What characterizes men who, like Callen, and Anthony and Kyle, have found the strength to carry on, and move forward, in the face of trauma? Central to their effective adaptation, such men have created, or rediscovered, a new framework of life's meaning in the context of HIV and AIDS. This framework offers keys that are crucial to fending off potential despair and meaninglessness: a coherent worldview, a sense of purpose, psychological stability, emotional vitality, and positive self-regard. I have come to identify eight characteristics that seem to typify such men:

- They believe they have the power, and the responsibility, to shape the meaning of their lives, especially their HIV infection.
- They fully admit the reality of their infection, but still maintain a capacity to distance themselves from AIDS and see it as an abstraction.
- They have discovered something in facing HIV or AIDS that unlocks a special quality within themselves.
- They feel a sense of kinship with other gay or HIV-positive men.
- They have a more "here-and-now" time focus.
- They believe in an afterlife, or other ongoing symbolic existence.
- They behave altruistically.
- They can tolerate the paradox, and the tension, of contradictory beliefs and feelings regarding HIV and AIDS.

Let's look at these in more detail.

Personal Control and Free Will

Perhaps the most basic underlying trait of men who have successfully forged meaning out of HIV and AIDS is a belief that people have choice or free will in ascribing meaning to their fate. The fact of HIV infection may be undeniable and irreversible, but what to do with this information, how to make use of it and live with it, is solely within a person's sphere of control.

This attitude was exemplified by Kyle, with words I quoted at the beginning of this chapter:

I know that I'm not getting away from this. It's real, it's here, inside, and how I choose to deal with it is key. . . . I've never had a very strong sense that I could get rid of this [HIV], heal myself that way, but I *do* have a strong sense that I can heal myself spiritually and emotionally.

Kyle knows that the *fact* of HIV infection is beyond his control, but its *meaning* is not. The one is a given, the other must be discovered. Being infected may seem horrible, unfair, even cataclysmic—but no amount of wishing or hoping is going to take it away. "It's real, it's here—how I choose to deal with it is key."

This opinion was not unusual among men with this style. Anthony said, "It's up to me to accept what's happening in my life or not." Roberto, the most robustly optimistic of the lot, said several times, "I think it's all how you look at it." Lucas likened his HIV infection to a Job-like challenge from God, undesired but seeded with the potential to "use it in some way that's redeeming."

Like Lucas, many of these men also had strong spiritual beliefs, most often believing in God or a supreme being. For them, this was not a God who preordained people's fate and actions—that remained up to each of us.

What is gained by this view? Why is it helpful to see HIV as something ambiguous and subjective, open to interpretation? Perhaps the central value of this belief is that it can go a long way in restoring a balanced sense of agency and control in life. AIDS no longer looms as something massively and utterly uncontrollable. The medical impact of the virus may be ultimately out of your hands, but you can steer the psychological course of infection by your own attitudes and activities. Again, Kyle's words are helpful: "I'm probably not going to be dying anytime soon. I've got time here. What am I going to do with this time?"

In this view, people have the opportunity—and the responsibility—to make the most of their circumstances. It's possible to view HIV in a variety of ways, and up to each person to wrestle with the reality of his infection, come to terms with it, and continually negotiate what role HIV will have in his life.

Real Yet Not Real:
HIV as Fact and Abstraction

This characteristic has two components. First is the ability to admit the reality of HIV—and this may not be as easy as it sounds. Admitting the reality of HIV infection means saying to yourself, honestly and baldly, "AIDS is real. HIV is real. I am infected with HIV. I can't dream or wish it away." This is the ability to stare into a mirror, look at yourself steadily, and utter the words that you are infected. Kyle again: "It's real, it's here."

Yet admitting the reality of HIV infection is only part of the picture. At the same time, it's very helpful to see HIV and AIDS as not real, to be able to gain distance from it. Being able to regard AIDS as an abstraction can be quite adaptive.

Being able to remove yourself from concerns about AIDS, to find some helpful respite, can offer valuable protection from sinking into panic, dread, or depression. It can be a productive means of psychological escape from worries over illness or impairment. Listen to the threads of "denial" in the words of Roberto:

> HIV presents tough challenges, emotionally difficult ones, emo-tionally enriching ones. It's added a whole new dimension to my life. If I could assure the outcome, I think I actually could embrace it. If I could know that "Hey, you know what? This is going to turn out okay, I'm going to be all right, they're going to come out with a way to maintain this permanently," then I would feel, "Wow, HIV is really basically a good thing."

Alas, Roberto can't "assure the outcome." He can't know for sure that things will "turn out okay." But by walking the delicate line between accept-ing and rejecting the facts of his situation, he allows the "emotionally enriching" challenges of HIV to be as present in his life as the "emotionally difficult ones."

And it *is* a delicate line. How can we differentiate between a helpful ability to see AIDS as an abstraction and a more destructive, dysfunctional denial?[3]

Seeing AIDS as an abstraction is not the same as believing that you can change your situation by sheer will, or that you are not really infected. Nor is it a fantasy of magical exemption or invulnerability, even though it may be hard not to indulge such occasional thoughts. And seeing AIDS as an abstraction is not a *behavioral* denial. In other words, it doesn't lead to dan-gerous activity, such as unsafe sex, neglecting your health, or substance abuse. Any use of denial that leads to increased health risk, to yourself or others, is maladaptive.

Instead, adaptively maintaining the ability to see AIDS as an abstraction means being able to acknowledge fears and concerns without being overwhelmed by them. It's being able to step back from HIV, to view it from a distance. It's being able, at times, to take a psychological "vacation" from the worries and stresses of HIV. These stresses may not completely disappear, but they take a back burner. The heat is lowered from full boil to gentle simmer.

Many HIV-positive individuals talk about the value of denial—calling it "creative denial," "helpful denial," whatever. And they're right—in appropriate measure, what a wonderful, necessary tool denial is.

Leon captured this balance of seeing AIDS as real yet not real. He was a physician in a large metropolitan hospital and much of his work involved people with AIDS, particularly in its end stages. When he began his medical residency, he had only known he was HIV-positive for a few weeks. The news of his infection surprised and devastated him. He hadn't had high-risk sex since 1981, and even then only had a small number of risky contacts. He had assumed he was negative for many years, and took the antibody test in 1988 seeking to confirm this. It didn't.

Still reeling from his positive test result, the start of Leon's medical residency proved disastrous. With distressingly vivid recall, he spoke about his first day at the hospital:

> In my first group of patients was an AIDS patient who was my age, at the end of his life, completely conscious of what was going on, and dying one of the more unpleasant deaths that people with HIV disease die of—not that any of them are pleasant, but he had a bleeding disorder, a platelet disorder, and was bleeding from every orifice of his body. He knew he was dying. He was lying there, terrified, telling me how frightened he was. His eyes were wide open, he didn't want to die. This was in the first group of patients I saw, and I flipped out.

Leon could not help identifying with this man. He said he saw himself in that bed. Learning that many of his patients would be people with AIDS was too much for him. Two days later he reneged on his residency and left the hospital. Despite the years and money he had just put into medical school, he feared that, because of HIV, he could never muster the strength to complete his training.

One year later, however, Leon began his residency again. He returned to the same hospital, the same AIDS caseload. And somehow, during the intervening year, he had developed the necessary distance to resume working.

In fact, a complete turnabout occurred. After returning to his residency, Leon began to derive a tremendous sense of purpose from his sensitivity to, and skill with, patients with AIDS.

To accomplish this transformation, Leon needed to develop strategies to protect himself. He had to weaken his identification with his patients. Without denying the reality of his own infection, Leon developed the capacity to see AIDS from a distance, as an abstraction:

> I've managed to put a distance between them and me in that situation, because I don't think of myself as being that sick. I think of myself as infected, and I think of an HIV sick person as being sick, so I've managed to put a distance in that sense. That enables me to go on, and deal with it.

He added that what also allowed him to work was a symbolic, and deeply ironic, gesture: He wore rubber gloves.

> I still feel funny about the medical practice of wearing rubber gloves, because you can't get AIDS from touching someone. . . . It bothers me, but on the other hand it enables me to keep that detachment.

From one vantage point, Leon is relying heavily on defense mechanisms that interfere with the accurate perception of reality. He uses the defense of "rationalization" to distinguish between himself and his patients. He uses "dissociation" to foster a sense of detachment that keeps him from being fully present. Yet to think of Leon's functioning from this perspective clearly misses the point: how necessary and helpful to strike a balance between nearness and distance, between acceptance and denial!

Yet not all people who have found HIV to be a transformative experience rely on this capacity to see AIDS as an abstraction. Some hone an opposite strategy. They vigilantly refuse themselves any "false hope." They use a steadfast awareness of the harsh reality of AIDS to spur on the growth they have achieved.

For example, Kyle wanted to "get as close to the HIV beast as possible." He tried not to invoke his "creative denial" when discussing the possibility of his own death. Instead, he expressed both fear and a hope that he could meet it head on, to confront it and learn from it:

> I've never been particularly afraid of death and dying. . . . I don't think I would commit suicide, although I would reserve for myself the right to do so. But I think there's so much in a spiritual dimension to be experienced by death and disintegration and letting go that I'm kind of more interested in that than in ending pain. But it will be very hard for me to confront a real disability. I'm very active, and hideously vain, and it would be hard for me to accept lesions, and having to spend a long time in bed. I'm going to have to work real hard to let go.

Similarly, when Anthony spoke of what he saw as the inevitability of developing AIDS, he neither shied away from, nor obsessively focused on, frank talk about death. In his usual style, he addressed the topic bluntly:

> I can't say, through most of this process, that I thought much about death other than to be afraid of it. It's only in the past two years, when my T-cells began to drop, that I've given serious consideration to the fact that I'm going to get sick and die soon, probably. . . . So in the past two years, death has come a lot closer. I'm trying to confront it and face it head on . . . I'd like to put myself around it physically more, because you see how death is just shunted aside in so many ways. It happens in hospitals, you don't see it, physically you don't have to confront it—of course, I also think I'd like to have barbiturates on hand, so I could cheat.

The Feeling of "Specialness"

For some men, HIV moves beyond being a burden to tolerate, a hardship begrudgingly accepted. It yields unexpected rewards through the difficult struggle of accepting its impact.

The ongoing process of coming to terms with HIV can unleash or reawaken previously dormant traits, talents, or strengths. HIV becomes a catalyst to discover internal resources that had never before been put to the test. Accepting the reality of being infected can act as a special key, opening previously unknown doors into the structure of identity—doors to rooms that hold valuable, perhaps long-forgotten treasures.

These treasures can vary. Maybe it's the knowledge that you are a stronger person than you thought. Perhaps it's a long-lost ability to act silly or frivolous—abandoning self-imposed, and culturally maintained, constraints of adulthood. Perhaps it's learning that you are an effective public speaker, a passionate activist, a truer friend, a more responsible and appreciative mate. Perhaps it's a deepening awareness, subtle but powerful, of your own courage.

Or perhaps it's a new ability to harness emotional struggles into powerful creativity. Coping with the turbulence and intensity of HIV has inspired in many a brilliant, elegiac creativity that might otherwise find no voice.

Art is often a conduit for emotion too raw to be confined to everyday language. Many gay men have funneled the grief that surrounds us—individually, collectively—into artistic works of passion and urgency. These outpourings strive to express an otherwise unspeakable pain, to gain mastery over the horror and incomprehensibility of it all.

But these creations also represent, for many artists, writers, and dancers (as well as businessmen, accountants, and lawyers) a self-expression deeper and more passionate than any previous creativity. AIDS, like any great despair, may don the cloak of Muse.

In other words, the strong jolt of HIV may propel someone in directions of inner discovery and productivity that would otherwise go untraveled. Leon's pride in being a good "AIDS doctor" captures this aspect of Transformation: "I know I'm a hell of a lot better at dealing with AIDS patients than almost any of my fellow house staff, and most of the attending doctors."

A Sense of Community

Connection to others is often a key aspect of transformative growth. As we've already seen, many men feel a sense of deep pride, even passion, regarding the gay community's accomplishments in facing AIDS. They have developed a deeper, surer sense of their own gay identity—a lessening of internalized homophobia, more comfort being out, a strengthening of feeling at home with gayness in themselves and others. Such sentiments were exemplified by Anthony, with words quoted at the chapter's beginning.

Anthony felt both a unique kinship with other HIV-positive men and a heightened affirmation of his own gay identity:

> One of the most positive experiences of my life recently has been my Body Positive group. Ten gay men who are HIV-positive—two with AIDS, others with other problems, others just HIV and doing pretty well, and we all look very much forward to getting together. We have a camaraderie and bonding which is unique in my life, wonderful and really supportive. There's an easiness in that room, and a liking of each other, which is really loving.

He returned to this theme frequently:

> There's going to be a lot of positive stuff that comes out of this. Gay people can now say "We" as a people in a way that we could-n't before this happened. I think we've responded to it. For me, the meaning of AIDS is going to be a lot of maturity on the part of the gay community. We're going to be healthier as a community than we were before. We're going to be more concerned about each other, and taking our lives as gay people more seriously.

Kyle viewed belonging to the gay community as an important vehicle for, and container of, his grief over AIDS losses. He spoke about attending a recent funeral for a friend:

> That was a real grieving experience for me, a wonderful opportu-nity to just let go. I cried and cried and cried, I cried like there was no end to it. . . . There was a collectiveness about it. I looked around and I knew just about everybody who was there, and I knew a lot of them to be infected themselves. A lot of families were there, and so it plugged me in at a lot of levels: there was the gay family, there was the nuclear family, kids, beautiful flowers, exquis-ite music, everything.

Community membership can take various forms—social, political, reli-gious, therapy or self-help based. Like many other men, Eugene connected his sense of belonging with a political pride in being out, both as gay and as HIV-positive:

It's very important that people come out as being positive whenever circumstances will allow, or whenever they have the guts, or whenever it's important to them. . . . I don't want to downplay my involvement [in the AIDS movement]. I want it to flow, and I don't want the feeling that I have to hold back on something I don't feel responsible for, or that it means anything negatively about me personally. I shouldn't apply the standards any differently than if I had leukemia or cancer.

A "Here and Now" Focus

HIV can lead to a changed awareness and appreciation of time. Developing a "here-and-now" focus allows for a greater capacity to appreciate life in the moment. It tempers the pain of real losses from the past and minimizes anxiety about the uncertainty of the future.

Part of acclimating to life with HIV is accepting the possibility of a foreshortened life or diminished future. This a source of great mourning —to some extent, a process that is unavoidable, necessary, and a precursor to deeper growth. For some people, this mourning eclipses all other aspects of their experience. Ruminating over the past and fearing for the future obscures any ability to live in the present.

However, some men also report a countervailing attitude. They mourn, but all is not sadness: Facing mortality becomes an impetus to accomplish goals or partake in activities that would otherwise be delayed. Leon captured this attitude:

This is it, you know, moment to moment, and trying to enjoy it, every moment. I'm not always successful, but I feel—not quite a pressure, but a strong sense that this is the only time we have, not next week, but now. Get everything you can out of living: do what you want to do, enjoy it. This feels like a positive thing, not a desperate thing—trying to treasure what's happening right now.

Similarly, Lucas also spoke about how HIV had significantly altered how he thought about time:

I'm much more aware of time passing, how I spend time, and taking time for myself to let myself live. I've always been so sched-

uled and on a timetable, pushing hard—that's been the story of
my life. HIV has introduced the other side, which is take time to
enjoy this moment, this day, don't push so hard doing all these
things you don't want to be doing.

He gained a new appreciation of time as embodied in nature:

I'm much more aware of seasons. I like being outdoors, and sometimes I think it's weird, here I am, 40 years old and just now realizing strawberries are here in the first two weeks of June.

Believing in an Afterlife

Many men with this style derive solace from contemplating a death that is
not absolutely finite. Whether they believe in a very specific concept of
heaven or reincarnation, or hold a more general conviction that some
unknown but peaceful spiritual plane follows this existence, this belief
becomes a powerful strategy for meaning. This may be true even for men
who do not embark on a broader spiritual journey.

How does believing in an afterlife connect to personal growth? Such
beliefs temper the indescribable loss, fear, and mystery that color the
serious contemplation of our own dying. Believing in an afterlife plays an
important role in maintaining life's meaning because it alters the finality of
death. And by altering the meaning of death, a person can begin reascribing meaning to life.

In other words, believing in an afterlife allows us to hope, despite HIV
and AIDS, that a part of us will remain alive after death. Alive, perhaps, to
enter into a deeper plane of spiritual energy, or to join beloved others who
have also died, or to fulfill our deep unconscious yearning of continuing to
exist. Believing in an afterlife allows us to strive for immortality.[4]

Fantasies of immortal life are deeply embedded in our unconscious.
They tap into primal concerns regarding annihilation and existence, being
and not-being. They typically operate far from day-to-day awareness, yet
their influence filters into the more mundane world of how we conduct our
lives. In fact, such fantasies may lie beneath many of our activities and
behaviors, even when those activities seem to be guided by less mysterious
or ephemeral needs.

For example, we've already touched on many benefits of a sense of
communal belonging: feelings of solidarity, comfort, and empowerment,

access to new information, diversion from inner ruminations, outlets for humor and worry, emotional support. Yet feeling part of a community also transcends these everyday concerns. It is a primary vehicle for our unconscious striving for immortality.

By strengthening one's communal identity as a gay man, the bonds a person develops surpass the limits of a specific friendship, a specific time. These bonds inseparably join someone with a life force that will be perpetuated beyond his death. Belonging to a community helps feed our deep wish that part of us will remain present after our own absence, that we will have achieved a symbolic immortality. This may be particularly relevant for gay men, in that most of us do not have children—a primary avenue through which many people address this deep unconscious striving to continue living on.

Let's return to Kyle. Kyle's HIV infection led him to a more spiritually oriented worldview, as well as to employment in an AIDS service organization. Recall that he derived enormous value (and meaning) from his work with individuals coping with the first shock and crisis of learning about their infection:

> Early on, I saw myself as an instrument: I've survived, there's something that I can help other people with here. This is my way of integrating what's happened to me, as well as integrating myself into a larger community. . . . At my most arrogant, in these groups that I lead, it's almost like I'm an initiator, or an elder for these men who have just learned they're positive. It's a wonderful feeling and I watch myself carefully so I don't abuse it, but I think, this is a rite of passage and I'm their initiator in a way. I'm one of the first people they see who's made some personal meaning out of being HIV positive, and that's my wish for them, that they make their own meaning out of it. . . . In the work that I do, I feel a sense of real connectedness with those men.

Kyle does not speak specifically in terms of "immortality." He does not work for the conscious reason of keeping a part of himself "alive." Yet a close look at his words also reveals this additional layer of meaning, along with the "real sense of connectedness" he feels with others.

Kyle expresses gratification at being the "initiator" of these men. He is an "elder" leading them into "a rite of passage." He sees himself as part of an ongoing ritual; he has something to offer, to teach, to be taken in by the group participants. He holds something unique that will be transmitted to others—so that when he has initiated them, it is no longer his alone. In some way, a part of him is being passed on, and kept alive, in other individuals.

Anthony's words, too, reveal his hope for symbolic immortality. His conviction in Christ's resurrection, literally and metaphorically, addresses the topic rather directly. Even more, Anthony's afterlife beliefs cannot be separated from his individual and communal identity as a gay man. In powerful and haunting words, he shared with me his wish for what might happen after his death. He conjured an image redolent with notions of immortality, spirituality, mystery, and gay brotherhood:

> I've heard, and this might be my fantasy, that at the cathedral at St. John of the Divine, the crucifix that dominates the apse is a columbarium, a relic or container of ashes of the dead. I've heard that it's mostly a container of ashes of people who have died of AIDS, and I love the idea that if I die, my ashes could go there and be part of that cross with other gay people. I like the idea of being buried with other victims of this epidemic. I don't want us to be forgotten as individuals or as a community who went through some spectacular suffering.

This striving for immortality is also part of what fuels art. The act of creation goes beyond expressing the anguish and bewilderment that can otherwise find no words: It is meant to reach beyond the moment, to last. In the context of AIDS, or any great sorrow, art is a vehicle to commemorate, to witness, to offer testimony of what has happened. It is meant to transcend.

Interestingly, many people who believe in an afterlife—either in facing their own mortality or grieving over a loved one—state that they *choose* to subscribe to this belief. A patient of mine comes to mind, a man coping with the death of his partner of many years. In his efforts to contain his grief, he commented, "I don't know if there is a heaven. But I tell myself there is one, and that Mitch is there."

Once again we enter the province of illusion. A heavenly afterlife may exist, it may not. Regardless, believing so brings comfort. How remarkable that people can create a belief, acknowledge that it may be a fiction, yet still use it to seek solace or meaning in their travails!

Altruism

For many men for whom HIV has led to personal growth, altruism has become a regular component of their lives. Kyle's devotion to assisting less experienced HIV-positive men, Leon's special attention to AIDS patients, Eugene's commitment to battling social inequities—all involve altruism. Similarly, Lucas, the minister, reflected on how his HIV infection had made him more compassionate and better able to empathize with the plight of others: "It's helped a great deal in my ability to enter people's places of pain and brokenness."

What are the benefits of altruism? It is more than an abstract concept: It involves actually *doing* something. Altruism bridges the gap between feeling compassion and acting compassionately, between a desire to help and actually pitching in. Praise and public recognition may offer secondary reinforcers, but most often one's good deeds go unsung. And even when it is received, praise may not even be as meaningful as the internal sense of finding value in giving. Altruism can be a helpful and productive way to regain a sense of personal control and meaning in an overwhelming situation.

Altruistic behavior takes many forms: direct service care, fund-raising, donating *pro bono* professional services, helping a friend above and beyond the call of duty. The specific activity need not be as relevant as simply doing something.

Altruism goes hand-in-hand with other characteristics of Transformation. Behaving altruistically often reflects, and strengthens, a sense of communal identity: The act of giving leads to a greater feeling of membership and belonging. (Altruistic behavior often feels as if it is "giving back," or reciprocating something that has already been received.) And altruism also helps satisfy our unconscious wishes for immortality—part of giving of ourselves is the hope that something will be passed along to survive.

This response to adversity is not unique to HIV. Altruism has been associated with psychological well-being among Holocaust survivors and others who have lived through "massive death" experiences.[5] It is a strategy trauma survivors often use to find meaning in their plight.[6] We can see this in how bereaved or traumatized individuals may become involved in work or causes related to the specific illness or traumatic event that affected them.

Tolerating Paradox

Finally, men with this style tend to see AIDS as a catalyst for significant personal growth *and* as an agent of irreparable, massive loss. HIV yields a bittersweet harvest of love and sorrow. Their growth does not turn an invisible eye to their loss.

These men have developed the capacity to tolerate the uncertainty of their situation and manage the ambiguity of holding contradictory thoughts, beliefs, and feelings. They live in a world where paradox, the essential union of opposites, registers as more "true" than believing this *or* that, one thing or another.

Leon, the physician, saw HIV as both a catalyst for personal growth and a harbinger of incomprehensible loss. He was living what he felt was a richer, more focused life. His medical skills were uniquely strengthened by his compassion for people with AIDS. He relished his newfound ability to "treasure" his relationship with Michael, his partner of nine years.

But Leon's sense of loss was equally profound as his hard-earned growth. This was voiced in his anxiety-ridden fears of death and his resentment at the timing of his positive test result. Leon grew up in an alcoholic, physically abusive family. At 19, he attempted suicide. At 23, he joined AA to overcome his own alcohol and multi-drug addiction. The following year, he began taking courses at a community college. After the financial and emotional "ordeal" of putting himself through ten straight years of education, he found out he was HIV-positive three days before his thirty-fourth birthday—and three weeks before his graduation from medical school.

Perhaps Eugene, more than any of the other men I spoke with, exemplified the ability (or perhaps the need) to tolerate the paradoxes of life amid AIDS. His lifelong involvement in progressive social activism was central to his self-identity. He saw himself, primarily, as "a community organizer." Since coming to terms with his own HIV infection—which followed a lengthy depression after learning the news—he had channeled his activism and commitment to social change into the AIDS movement.

For Eugene, HIV had led to much growth. At 45, he previously felt alienated from mainstream gay culture: "I always had a few radical gay male friends—but they were also poets." He now felt more integrated into, and accepting of, the world of gay men. He had formed "lasting friendships" with gay men toward whom he once felt defensively "superior." He rejoined a Catholic church, and emotionally offered his first confession in 35 years.

He felt "more moderate," "more organized," "wiser," "smarter," and "more mature." His unpaid volunteer work for an AIDS organization required more time than a full-time job, and as much commitment.

But equally vivid was Eugene's sense of contamination and punishment. On the one hand, in words already quoted, he talked about being proud of who he was, and the need to be publicly identified as HIV-positive:

> It's very important that people come out as being positive when-ever circumstances will allow, or whenever they have the guts, or whenever it's important to them. . . I don't want the feeling that I have to hold back on something I don't feel responsible for, or that it means anything negatively about me personally.

Yet, on the other hand, he saw AIDS as "an embarrassment" that "set everything back: It's exposed our dirty linen." AIDS had bared to the world secrets about "bathhouses and harnesses and tit rings"—aspects of gay life that were, he had come to think, "sleazy, silly, and a little gross." Eugene was a man with a tremendous ability to energetically and creatively enliven his world, and actively strive to make sense of his situation—but this activity served dual purposes, making him feel both more proud and more ashamed of who he was.

Lucas struggled to capture the paradoxical and tenuous balance between HIV-initiated growth and loss. I asked him—as I asked all the men—if he had found any beneficial aspects of being HIV-positive. He shared both his own sense of personal growth and his rage at those who see such growth in a naive and global manner:

> There have definitely been positive aspects, but it would be too easy, too simple to say "Oh yeah, there's a lot of good things about HIV." I can't do that: There *are* good things about it, but first I have to acknowledge how horrible it is, how bad it is, and how much I wish it wasn't in the world, not only just in me. . . . I get very irritated when I hear simplistic "feelings" that are very posi-tive about it—"It's wonderful, HIV is just wonderful in my life." I want to slap those people around. Fuck you, it's positive: It's also horrible! . . . Half the universe is getting thrown away there. Let's acknowledge that other half, how shitty it is, how horrible it is,

how bad it is. So with that said, yes, there's a lot of good things that happened.

"So with that said, yes . . ." Lucas believes that HIV has yielded benefits, but only embedded in a larger reality of tragedy and pain. He seems to feel he dare not overemphasize his growth, for this would diminish the horror. But neither can he ignore it, for that would invalidate the truth of his experience. The indescribable contradiction of what he feels resides outside the realm of language. Words cannot do it. Growth and loss together, intertwined, one and the same—what utter, irreducible paradox.

―――――――――

These, then, are some characteristics of men who have met the enormous challenge of integrating HIV and AIDS into a new, growth-oriented framework of meaning. These themes are general guidelines and commonalities, not fixed or necessary traits. They stem from several representations of HIV—HIV as a catalyst for personal or spiritual growth, increased belonging, and the paradoxical acceptance of irreparable loss.

When I first sorted through the interviews and identified men who fit this style of adaptation, I hoped to find patterns that connected them. The question that had stayed with me for years resurfaced: Where is the meaning, for me, for others? How comforting it would be if I could discern some easy formula or clues that captured the essence of transformative growth. Did these men bear similarities, in terms of their exposure to others with HIV, their physical health, their pre-AIDS life history?

That seemed not to be the case. For some of them, AIDS had so far remained at the periphery of their lives. They had not experienced any AIDS-related deaths and had minimal contact with ill individuals. But others were drenched in loss. Kyle's lover Frank had died, and Anthony had seen the deaths of over 25 men he knew. Lucas had not only lost several close friends to AIDS, but had taken on the repeatedly painful challenge of officiating at their, and other AIDS-related, funerals.

Some of these men were in good health, with no outward signs of immune difficulty other than awareness of their seropositivity. Yet Stan (whom I discussed in HIV as relief) had been hospitalized with a near lethal bout of pancreatitis, incurred as a reaction to an experimental drug, and Anthony, who had known of his immune deficiency since 1981, had a bleak T-cell count of 57. And while many had never faced life situations as stressful as their current infection, Leon and Roberto had grown up in alcoholic, abusive households.

Some were in satisfying relationships, others weren't. Some liked their jobs, others didn't. In other words, other than their ability to forge a path for life's meaning in the context of HIV, this was not a homogeneous lot.

But they did share some things. For almost all, the process of maintaining meaning was an ongoing journey, always changing, always developing, with many twists and turns. Almost all of them spoke of a time, earlier in their infection, of depression and anxiety. Anthony, whose pivotal turnabout came with joining Alcoholics Anonymous, had spent several years having unsafe sex and flirting with suicide. Leon assumed he would never have the courage to return to medicine. Almost all went through expected period of devastation after first learning of their infection.

And by the time my life intersected with theirs, each had learned how to fortify himself against a sorrow and bitterness that could have quite easily gained the upper hand. By struggling to embrace the paradox of joy and loss; by striving to achieve immortality symbolically through art, spirituality, community, or love; by spinning a benevolently self-deceptive life narrative that at once gave AIDS full due and ignored its presence, men such as Kyle, Anthony, Lucas, and Eugene resurrected the essence of a meaningful life.

These were not superheros or ideals. These were real men, with admirable strengths but also with difficulties, quirks, and frailties that are all too human. Meeting with them was inspiring and humbling—because of their impressive resilience, I was left to marvel even more about the courage some people demonstrate in the face of hardship. And as I tried to piece together what they shared, I recognized how much of the journey must be self-discovered rather than dictated. How can you teach someone (in psychotherapy, in friendship, from a course or a book) to embrace paradox, to forge symbolic immortality, to strike a balance of deceiving and not deceiving oneself?

Transformation requires initiative; perhaps *that* can be taught. Behaving altruistically, seeking out kinships with others, developing (and acting on) new priorities, making time for activities that would otherwise be delayed, testing the boundaries of what can be controlled and what must be accepted—all these take initiative. A person cannot be a passive participant in the process of finding meaning in life. It doesn't magically descend from the heavens in full regal garb.

But initiative is not enough. There is a difference between surviving adversity—an admirable feat in itself—and transforming it into a catalyst for growth. Transformation may require alchemy at more private, and more primitive, levels of the psyche. It may only be possible when we make inroads into mastering the deep, instinctual fear of death that lurks within our unconscious. A person need not overcome that fear (is this even possible?), but perhaps only glance at it without shying away, acknowledge it, open himself up to it in a more searing and exposing way than before.

It is the terrible immanence of death that fuels AIDS' threat to living meaningfully. In the face of such inestimable loss, glimpsing death's truth may be a necessary midwife in the rebirth of a life of meaning.

Some accomplish this—quietly, heroically, impressively. But for many others (positive and negative) the devastation of HIV has been too great. AIDS has destroyed their ability to see the world as meaningful. They experience what I call Rupture, the next style we will explore.

5

Rupture: The Shattering of Meaning

Victor: I couldn't have written this, I don't think anybody could have thought this up. If anyone had . . . people would have said it's too fantastical, it's impossible that this kind of stuff could happen. People don't have lives like this, people don't have these things happen to them.

Ron: It just shouldn't be—it's a cheat, a terrible cheat. . . . This is something that I did not anticipate happening to me and my friends. We all lived in the bubble of modern medicine, there were more and more antibiotics and drugs to take care of things. People didn't die young anymore unless they were hit by a bus or went down in a plane crash, it just didn't happen. AIDS has remade everything.

Howard: It's unbelievable to me that all these young men are dead or dying . . . I don't understand. There's so little time to do anything, so little that can be counted on. . . . It makes me astonished by how much suffering is in the world. There is so much pain going on, and my exposure to AIDS and people dying somehow makes it all more real to me.

With its relentless barrage of illness, loss, and grief, AIDS has the devastating power to shatter peoples' views of life as meaningful. In the style of adaptation I call Rupture, a person bears the full brunt of HIV's despair and trauma. For these men, grief is too weighty to be countered by hope. Sorrow may cut too deep to allow for stability, much less growth.

Here loss, not growth, is key. Gone is the comfort of a safe and orderly world. Gone is the expectation of a lengthy lifespan. Gone is the soothing and helpful illusion of immortality. Gone, often, are the very lovers and friends with whom one would otherwise seek shelter from the steadily mounting losses. In one dire flash—or, more commonly, in painful, inexorable increments of loss—AIDS has robbed these men of the inner beliefs and external bonds on which they based their lives. It has unceremoniously yanked the rug of meaning out from under their feet.

Rupture results from losing your prior framework for understanding the world, with no new beliefs to take their place. Victor and Ron are examples of this style of adaptation.

Victor: "I'm saturated in death"

Victor was the most emotionally flamboyant man I interviewed. In the course of the several hours we spent together he ricocheted from despair, to rage, to venom, to humor. He could not alight on any one mood or thought for long without restlessly flitting someplace else. One moment he spoke with the serenity of a Zen monk; the next he buzzed like a pinball machine with too many bells and lights.

In fact, it is only through contradictions that I can adequately describe Victor. They were everyplace: in his looks, his life history, his verbal style.

Victor is 42 years old. When we met he was clad all in black (T-shirt, jeans, boots) with a shaved head and numerous earrings—a look emphasizing both an enticing sexuality and the premature haggardness of his face. Professionally, he was a licensed Shiatsu massage therapist, but he had hop-scotched around jobs quite a bit—restaurants, theater, dance, various other activities here and there. His voice was as mercurial as his mood, raspy one moment (like a bald, black-clad Lauren Bacall), a soft teasing purr the next. And no matter his emotional state, he described it in extreme terms: "100%," "absolute," "the worst," "the best." He ended many statements by exclaiming "period!" as if unaware of the dramatic force with which he had already delivered most of what he said.

No doubt Victor's frenzied interpersonal manner long preceded any impact of the epidemic—this was not a style that seemed caused, in any major way, by AIDS. But I think his dizzying restlessness also related to HIV. His manner seemed to reflect both a fiercely impassioned approach to life and an enraging inability to make sense of, or tolerate, what his world had become.

The word "alienation" cropped up repeatedly in Victor's talking. Feeling alienated had been a primary aspect of his experience throughout life:

> I never fit in when I was growing up, in any of the environments I lived in. I never felt comfortable—but that hasn't changed a hell of a lot, either. I still don't necessarily feel like I fit in, nor am I accepted or comfortable. More so than before, perhaps, but there's still a part of me that feels very much like an outsider to everything, to it all. The image is *The Man Who Fell to Earth*. When that film came out, I identified with it 100%. I feel like I was just dropped on this planet.

With HIV, Victor's sense of alienation has grown stronger, both from straight society and within the gay world:

> Automatically, immediately, you've been set aside, you've been segregated, you've been labeled something "different than" . . . even within the gay community I feel different, separated at times because I'm positive, they're negative. . . . That changes how you feel about feeling comfortable in the world, and I don't already feel comfortable in the world, so it makes me feel even less welcome—I felt a lot more welcomed in the world in 1981 than 1991; in 1991, I feel basically, the attitude is "It's all right if you drop dead, we really won't miss you."

Victor moved to Manhattan from the Connecticut suburb where he grew up in the 1970s, participating in the fast-paced, cutting-edge New York gay life of the time. He "traveled in a lot of the leather/Levi kind of crowd, the Mineshaft, the fast lane of New York City." He loved the hedonism of that world, celebrating the spiritual and sexual "exploration," pushing the limits of conventional mores. It also provided him, more than at any other point in his life, with a sense of belonging.

Prior to the epidemic, Victor felt as if his life had already bottomed out and that he had recovered. In 1980, he got sober. Victor's drinking and drug problems were extreme; he believes that alcohol and pills might have killed him had he not gotten them under control. He looks back on gaining sobriety as one of the great turning points and accomplishments of his life.

At the time, Victor had no way of anticipating how gaining sobriety would foreshadow, as it did, the difficult task of facing AIDS. Getting sober provided him with a model for coping with major difficulty; it solidified for him a belief in the possibility of change. These would be helpful assets when the deluge hit.

Still, sobriety could not prepare him for the staggering number of deaths in his world that began a few years later. Friends, acquaintances, sex buddies began dying in quick succession. The number kept on growing. By the time his lover Alan died in 1987, he felt depleted of the strength or desire to carry on.

> I've stopped counting [deaths], and I stopped counting when Alan died. At that point it was about 30. I have sat down on occasion and written lists, and try to think; I inevitably forget people and then it will come to me, and now I don't even try to do that anymore, because I can't. After Alan died, that was a very significant loss, I don't think that I will ever lose anything more significant. So the rest of the deaths, it's not that they don't matter, but [starts crying]—that was a good place to stop counting.

Victor's cumulative losses compound and echo one another, making each additional loss more difficult to assimilate:

> There's a variety of types of losses, in the sense of lovers, boyfriends, people that are very close to me, and then there are friends, acquaintances, and clients, I lose a lot of clients. Every time someone I've been close to, intimate, sexual with, whatever, dies, the whole thing has to be replayed through, in some way. That's begun to take its toll on me; I find it difficult to go through that again and again and again. There's a part of me that shuts down, and I don't like that, but if I face it, I can't function.

In many ways, Victor has coped well with AIDS' omnipresence in his life, and with his own HIV infection (confirmed by an antibody test two years prior to our meeting). He has not returned to drinking. He continues working as a massage therapist. He has had to curtail many activities in his life because of fatigue, but HIV has allowed him to be "totally expansive" about himself . . . "this isn't a dress rehearsal."

Yet as our interview wove in and out of his many moods, it became increasingly clear that what simmered beneath Victor's theatrical style was a staggering sense of loss. It was this pain that kept him buzzing around, a constant fluttering to avoid settling into the true brunt of his anguish.

> I don't know if I really want to get old. There's not a lot of people left in my life, and I'm worn out trying to make new friends, have them get sick and die. I don't want to be old and alone, I don't know what value there is in surviving for the sake of just surviving. I think, most of the time lately, death might be a welcome relief from what this is, what life has become.

He could find no words to comprehend the magnitude of AIDS' impact and presence. It amazed him that life continued unaffected for so many people:

> I couldn't have written this, I don't think anybody could have thought this up. If anyone had thought it up or written it, and people read it, they would have said it's too fantastical, it's impossible that this kind of stuff could happen: people don't have lives like this, people don't do these things, people don't have these things happen to them. . . . There will be times when I will be on the subway, walking on the street, and I'll look around. Assuming everyone I look at is straight—which is a stupid point of view—I'll think, "Jesus guys, look at this, you're all running around like fucking maniacs. If you only had an inkling, if you only knew a little bit of what I've gone through, what I've experienced, somehow I think it would change what you're all running around here about."

Victor's style of emotional intensity also extended to how he talked about death. More so than any of the other men with whom I met, Victor discussed death with an immediacy—an intimacy—that offered scant solace or detachment.

Death was all around him. It was in his raw grief for his lover, in his cumulative pain for many lost friends and acquaintances, in his fantasies of suicide. It was in his black garb (which fit his persona so well, I assume he wore it all the time). It was in the premature thinning face, in his pained eyes.

More than anyplace else, death's presence was in the impassioned, almost reverential, tone with which he spoke about his contact with dying people. Here, in his mercurial presentation, Victor seemed most monklike, most spiritual. In his work as a massage therapist, his clientele included many people with AIDS, particularly those in the end stages of life:

> There are times it's very scary. . . . I'll be in the midst of doing it and for an instant, it will totally freak me out what I'm doing. But then it seems like the most, the only, natural thing I could be doing. It's difficult, and it's painful. At times it's like I'm saturated in death. But it's a tremendous honor to be allowed to come into someone's life right before they die, it's a very altering experience.
>
> I just worked with a man who died two weeks ago. He was fortunate in the sense that he was very wealthy, and had part of his home set up like a hospital room: hospital bed, IV, so he could die at home. . . . There wasn't much left of his person. You don't really do massage [with dying people] because there's not much left of their body, you just do touch. . . . Between the times that I worked with him, his body, at first, was holding on to everything. But the last time I worked with him, five days before he died, he had let go significantly, and wanted to let go more. In doing the work, I verbally encourage a person to "let go, let go," and that message goes through very deeply. Most clients, I'm talking about letting go of a certain amount of muscle tension, but the same message gets through to someone a couple of hours away from dying, or a couple of days. It's all right to let go.

As Victor continued talking, he entered a reverie of sorts. His tone grew hushed, far away. In describing such vivid images of working with a dying person, the roles became muddied. He began speaking less to me, more to himself. It was now his death intruding into his thoughts, his dying:

> In this intimate work I do with people, I see myself, it's like it's me on the table, and I hope—people will see me upset when I've lost a client, and say, "Why don't you just not do the work?," and it makes me very angry. My response is "How can I not do the

work?" Somebody has to do the work, and I'm glad somebody is doing the work. I hope that should I, when I, if I, it's like putting money in the bank. I hope there's somebody there to come and do that for me. That's a lot of how and what my life is about at this point—it's a lot about showing people how I want to be taken care of . . . so that they'll know and they'll see and they'll understand and they'll be able to do it in a way that's not scary and that's dignified, loving, all of those things.

By the end of our lengthy interview, I had the sense that Victor's immersion in loss, both his own bereavements and those of others, had indelibly bled into every aspect of his life. He sought and found escape from what he called "his ghosts" in temporary pursuits. He rallied against despair with humor, anger, and flamboyance. But he seemed depleted, or with only minimal reserves of strength. He was exhausted from so much grief and saw no reason to hope for the future. In his own words, he was a man "saturated in death."

Victor's despair was such that he compared AIDS to the Nazi Holocaust, and the Holocaust emerged as the more tolerable and benign of the two:

People say, this is what it's like to be in war. That may be a good analogy. Concentration camps may be a good analogy. But somehow all of those things have had the grace of a limit of time: a war lasts four years, or it lasts ten years, the concentration camps ended. This hasn't ended, it doesn't end. This doesn't end. . . .

Victor's response can be understood in terms of his personality style: his extreme view, and belief that his suffering is "the worst" and beyond others' understanding, reveal both grandiosity and narcissism. And Victor certainly did present himself in a rather grand and self-centered way. But so what? All that seems of secondary importance, compared with the enormity of his need to find meaning in his situation and his inability to do so.

Ron: "It just shouldn't be"

Ron looked older than his 44 years. Recent HIV-related health problems, and his still pressing grief for his lost lover, Robert, had aged him. His simple, utilitarian clothing—jeans and a flannel shirt, before they became faddish—no longer fit. They hung too largely on his frame. He was not very ill, but even on first meeting, he looked like a man whose life spirit had taken some battering.

Our interview got off on shaky footing. Within the first few minutes, Ron told me of Robert's death ten months previously. Perhaps I did not respond with enough sensitivity to his pain; perhaps his pain was such that no response would have been empathically adequate. Whichever it was, the first 40 minutes of our meeting had an antagonistic edge, absent from the other interviews. It seemed more a process of wrangling with one another than of building rapport.

Although Ron's sharp intelligence was apparent from the outset, his manner was pedantic and devoid of emotional resonance. I felt as if he were lecturing to me. When I asked him how HIV had affected his life, he gave a dry and obtuse answer about the cultural implications of AIDS. I tried probing further, gently, and got more of the same. Finally, feeling a little exasperated, I asked again, personalizing the question in a rather direct way: "How about *you*? How has AIDS or HIV affected *you*?"

He paused, and his emotional distance crumbled into tears. He began to speak slowly, with far less self-assurance. He articulated his words carefully, almost as if hoping to grasp onto them for support, or perhaps discover in them something previously unrevealed:

> How has it affected me? Well, there are a lot of people who are dead, and it shouldn't be—it just shouldn't be. Now, everyone dies, but not everyone dies at 45 and 30. [Long pause] It's the most serious disruption of my life that I have yet experienced. [Crying heavily] It steals the time that was rightfully ours, and there's no replacing that. There were things I thought I had more time to do, relationships that I thought I had more time to savor. That whole process has been foreshortened.

His tears chastened me. Why had I been so needlessly blunt? I should have realized all along: Our opening wrangle and Ron's pedantry had been a front. An understandable, and necessary, front. It probably helped him some. But it was paper thin, inadequate when charged with the monumental task of keeping his despair at bay.

As we continued talking, I learned that Ron felt inconsolably devastated by what AIDS had done to his life. His was a world of bewildering, senseless loss. He could no longer work, because he wearied easily and early onset neurological difficulties had affected his concentration. His losses were those more typical of extreme old age than of a man in his forties. And he found no meaning in any of what had befallen him.

Ron was raised in a small town in Missouri. He described his parents as "kind, well-meaning, unenlightened, rock-ribbed Republicans." The town was "not an environment that tolerated social deviation of any kind," so he resisted pressure to enter the family business and settle down. He moved away at 18, leaving for college in one city, and, eventually, graduate school for social work in another.

As I listened to Ron talk about his life prior to AIDS and HIV, it seemed that two central themes were primary in giving shape and purpose to his existence. One was the continual questioning (and frequent rejection) of social rules. He defined himself, rather proudly, as a person who defied social expectations. He saw adhering to conventional norms as "shallow." He dismissed the values of his parents and hometown as "stifling." Yet he was equally dismissive of conventions in the gay world, which he disparaged as "superficial." He said he labeled himself as gay, but mostly for political reasons; in theory and practice, he saw himself as bisexual. He felt no more sense of belonging in the mainstream world of gay men than he did in his hometown.

Second, related to this rejection of conventionality, Ron had always sought out a spiritual understanding of life: "For many years, I had a lot more experience of my spiritual being than I did of my physical being." His spiritual path focused on alternative channels — Eastern religions, hallucinogenic drugs, mystical texts. In the Eastern spirituality that informed his outlook on life, sex had been a key element of spirituality:

I believe that what sex is actually for . . . beyond reproduction . . . is that it's a ladder to god. I think what happens when people have significant sexual communication with one another is that the energies that we build upon, back and forth in a good sexual exchange, systematically work their way up through the chakras, leading to the frontal lobe and the cerebral cortex.

Ron's rejection of conventional norms influenced many of his life choices. He pursued social work as a career because of his beliefs in the value of community service. He experimented with several alternative living arrangements over the years—communes, communal households, living in a *menage à trois* with both a male and female partner. At another time, he lived in a household with seven other men, idealistically hoping to pioneer a new kind of gay male family.

AIDS entered into Ron's life in the early 1980s, and steadily hammered away over the next several years. First came the illness and death of an ex-lover. By 1985, he knew that both he and his then current lover, Robert, were infected. By 1988, all the men in his gay family had died except Robert and him. Then Robert died too. He was the only one left.

The loss of these close friends, lovers, and intimate partners became inseparably intertwined with Ron's concerns about his own early death:

> I thought I would have more time, and the company of those people who were dearest to me, to make greater sense of this. . . . It's given me a lot to cope with that is out of phase with my life. Ordinarily, at 44 I would not be going through the processes of mourning that I have been, a real sense of closing down that I've experienced in the past several years. This should have been the height of my career, but such as it is, it is.

Above all else, most distressing and painful for him was the death of Robert, whom he described as his "life partner":

> Robert's loss is the one I feel most grievously. [crying heavily] He was the love of my life. The others are people who touched me very deeply, and were able to give to me in very special ways and are absolutely irreplaceable, but the loss of someone with whom I'd shared so much intimacy, physical and otherwise, such as in the relationship with Robert—it's an order of several magnitudes greater than any loss I have ever experienced before, or hope to again.

Unfortunately, Ron's spiritual beliefs, which had been so crucial in giving his life meaning prior to AIDS, offered no help in his need to render some sense from his many losses. His religious ideas — difficult to integrate with daily life in the first place — had failed him. Perhaps this was because his spirituality had always been abstract rather than personal, providing him a model to think about life in general, but not to feel comfort in specific ways:

> I know that there are larger patterns of which we make up a part and that rarely, if ever, do we get much of an inkling of what that's about — occasionally epiphanies, peak experiences, that kind of thing, precious moments. So I know that that's true, that there's a higher truth. . . . But I don't believe that God, or the forces of the universe, whatever you want to use to describe those larger factors at work, is much involved at the personal level at all. . . . I don't think that our individual, or perhaps collective fate, is of concern to those larger forces.

So to some extent, Ron's spirituality still provided him some shreds of meaning. But it seemed to me incomplete, for it was a meaning that ignored *him*. His spiritual views offered him no solace, no compassion. Unlike Anthony, he had no sense of being divinely loved or held, of using spirituality to discover a place of belonging.

Ron's losses were immense. He had lost his lover, his friends, his work. When we met, Robert had been dead for just under one year; Ron's grief was still visceral and raw. No amount of spiritual searching, or rational inquiry, helped him make sense of what AIDS had done to his life. He hungered for some answer that would bring at least an explanation, if not a reason. He both believed and disbelieved that HIV resulted from governmental activity, malicious or accidental:

> My paranoid sensibility says this is the result of some bioengineering, some recombinant DNA stuff that got out of hand. Whether it was the CIA, or someone else in the government, who knows? We'll never know about that. But that's just my paranoid self; I suppose this is something that just came into existence.

For Ron, HIV meant mainly isolation and irreparable loss. His many losses were beyond his emotional wherewithal. I think his "paranoid sensibility" (whether accurate or not) stemmed from a profound longing to discover some reason, some understandable purpose or rationale, in the tragedy that his life and world had become. He needed some sense, some order, some respite from the grief and devastating sense of meaninglessness.

Ron was certainly not without strengths. He had intelligence, inner motivation, undeniable tenacity, and an admirable ability to follow his own path. His unconventional life choices did not hamper an ability to connect with other people. Even his prickly exterior no doubt came in handy.

But these resources could not compete with what he was up against. Ron's anger was useful, but it also had the false, childlike bravado of someone who knows, deep down, that he faces a power much greater than himself. He sniped and fought back with defiance, but what lurked behind his words was an agonizing sense of incredulity and sorrow. He intoned the same refrain over and over, like a mantra of protest against a broken law of justice: "It just shouldn't be."

For Victor and Ron, and other men similar to them, HIV has ruptured their previous view of the world as meaningful. The unfairness of AIDS colors most every aspect of life, everpresent, like a wound that can find no anodyne.

Beneath these men's despair is disbelief and a sense of betrayal. How could so monstrous a deviation from life's expectations occur? Who misled them into believing that life was fair, the world kind, the fates benevolent? How could God do this? How could this happen—how *dare* this happen, to me, to us? Perhaps more than sorrow, more than the pain of loss, the heart of Rupture is this jarring disillusionment. The beneficial illusions that may have given shape to life before no longer work.

Four of the men I spoke with—Ron, Victor, Howard, and Charles—demonstrated this response to HIV. For them, the combination of losses from AIDS and their own HIV infection had shorn away the fabric of beliefs on which they had based their lives. For each of the men, except Charles, the inability to find meaning in his situation, or the shattering of his previous life's meaning, was a conscious source of turmoil. They were hounded by unanswered, and perhaps unanswerable, questions: Why? Why me? Why gay men? Why AIDS? Why my friends and lovers?

Unlike the bittersweet gains of the men I described in Transformation, these men saw no beneficial aspects of HIV. Howard identified nothing positive. Ron at first tentatively suggested that HIV had been an impetus to further grapple with spiritual issues, but then backed down, deciding that "It's probably just the case that I'm trying to come up with something" because I had asked the question. Victor responded with his acerbic wit that "Yes, of course [there are benefits]—I get free theater tickets."*

Both Victor and Ron had already experienced physical impairments from HIV—a fact that cannot be disentangled from their psychological adaptation. Yet I don't think the presence or absence of actual debility is what most strongly determines HIV's impact on meaning. Anthony continued moving forward in life with 57 T-cells; Charles struggled to stay afloat with no discernible presence of ill health.

Perhaps more relevant than actual health, Rupture is most common in men whose main representations of HIV are irreparable loss and isolation. The presence of AIDS in their life, or in the world, is experienced as calamitous and unfair, with no sense of gain for counterbalance, no working through the loss to a place of paradoxical acceptance.

The isolation of these men often lacks a compensatory sense of increased belonging. Grief is always a lonely undertaking, but for these men there may be no glimmer of solace or meaning that others find in a community. It's not that their lives are necessarily devoid of contact: Ron attended an AIDS bereavement group and had the support of close friends; Howard and Charles had lovers; and Charles also had his daily 12-step meetings. But each felt isolated within these social structures. They believed something about their pain was beyond understanding. Despite the presence of others, each remained alone.

Howard, the art historian, found a metaphor for his sense of meaninglessness in art:

> Because of what I do for a living, I'm very aware of the notion of style. You simply watch one be supplanted by another, and another, and another, until you wait for them to depart: I don't get this one, so I'll go on to the next one. When you're dealing with lives . . . there has to be some meaning. It just can't be that people come in one door and they go out the other, like fads or styles.

Despite his disbelief that "it just can't be," Howard had no guiding understanding or explanation as to why "it" was. He dismissed religion as an option. Nor did he derive meaning from a sense of kinship with others.

---

*Some AIDS service organizations arrange for free theater tickets to individuals with HIV or AIDS.

In his eyes, he was isolated from white gay men because of his race, isolated from other black people because of his sexuality, and isolated from the other black gay men he knew because of his professional and economic standing. He had no community to call home.

How telling that Howard could have chosen to talk about art as something lasting or transcendent, as a process that imbues meaning, but instead highlighted a particular aspect of art history that mirrored his inability to find meaning in his losses: the impermanence or ephemerality of artistic styles.

Most men go through a period of something akin to Rupture in the early phases of dealing with being positive. In this regard, it is like a period of shock people typically experience in the immediate aftermath of a major loss or catastrophe. In presenting Rupture as an ongoing pattern of adaptation to HIV, I am not referring to this initial reaction. Instead, these are men for whom a sense of purpose or meaning does not rebound. Their framework of meaning remains shattered, or gets more distressed as time continues.

Like the other styles of adaptation, certain themes may be relevant to men with this response.

Unresolved Grief

Just as a belief in personal control or free will may form the bedrock of Transformation, unresolved grief is apt to be the primary determinant in Rupture. These men have usually experienced a dear loss, or several, from which they have not recovered. The inability to heal from this loss (or losses) halts the process of reestablishing meaning in life.

This simply may be cruel accrual. One additional loss, piled atop many, becomes too much to bear. But more often, the destruction of meaning comes from the death of someone very particular and dear—a loss "on an order of several magnitudes greater" than any other, to use Ron's words.

The deaths of Alan (Victor's lover) and Robert (Ron's lover) represent this type of bereavement. Both Victor and Ron had experienced many other losses, which they grieved and mourned. Yet as they told their life stories, it became clear that the loss of their lover was qualitatively different from their earlier (and later) losses, and much more damaging. Each was already struggling to maintain his stability in the face of AIDS and HIV; their lovers' deaths tilted the balance sadly into the direction of meaninglessness.

Not all deaths, or all grief experiences, destroy meaning. Kyle and Anthony both suffered tremendous losses, yet were able to reestablish a sense of purpose in their life. Why is it that some losses are so much harder to bear than others?

Researchers who study widowhood have examined this question. Some data suggest that two types of marriages are most likely to result in a complicated, entrenched, unresolved pattern of grief: those in which the widow felt very dependent on her husband, and those in which she had strong ambivalent feelings about him, but felt she could neither accept nor express her negative feelings.[1]

Can we apply these same studies to gay widowhood in the context of AIDS? Perhaps not, for a few key reasons. Heterosexual widowhood does not match the unique situation of gay lives and relationships. It does not speak to the reality of continual, multiple loss that AIDS has created in many of our lives. And most widows do not simultaneously face profound concerns regarding their own mortality while grieving their mate. So far, unfortunately, very little research has been conducted into our unique grief —the grief of gay men amid the multiple bereavements of AIDS.[2]

Yet with that said, there may be some parallels. Clearly—witness the difference between Kyle and Ron—some grief responses are more protracted and shattering than others. Some people rebound from loss relatively quickly, others not at all. How a gay man grieves his lover's death may well be influenced by issues of dependence, or ambivalence, or some other interpersonal factor central to a particular relationship.

And some folks may just be more sensitive to loss, regardless of the nature of their relationships. Shaped by biology, early life experience, or a combination of the two, they exhibit greater anxiety and fear in response to separation. Ron and Victor, and others who display this pattern of adaptation, may be predisposed to more intense and intractable grief reactions, to a heightened sensitivity to loss. For them, amid the general devastation of AIDS, a loss too dear can be the straw that breaks the camel's back. It echoes loudly and endlessly because there is too little else to cushion the sound of its reverberating pain.

With grief such as this, we see why believing in free will—a central feature of Transformation—isn't enough by itself. Ron certainly believed in free will, as did Victor, but neither could translate such belief into growth. For them, what good was thinking that people have the option of finding their own meaning in life when they had been robbed of such a crucial support?

Inability to Escape from Concerns about AIDS

Men with this style tend to have no respite from AIDS concerns. They lack the ability to see AIDS as "real yet not real." In contrast to some others, who are so defended against AIDS' impact that they ignore the real effects of HIV on their lives, these men do not have *enough* defense. They need more self-protection. They need more access to a denial that might assuage the bitterness of constant awareness.

For these men, the filter of HIV may become a lens through which everything is now seen. They cannot escape it. Victor saw AIDS everyplace —it not only defined the gay world he inhabited, but he also focused on its absence from the straight world. On subways or city streets, AIDS was still painfully present for him, seeing how it *wasn't* present for others. When Ron said AIDS had "remade everything," I imagine he was referring not only to the world around him but also his inner self, and the stripping away of necessary distance.

Men who have been affected by HIV in this manner need to move gingerly, for it is as if they walk on psychological egg shells. The most seemingly innocuous or mundane activity can immediately re-ignite a jarring awareness of rage or loss. Daily life may become one unending litany of intrusive reminders—reminders of AIDS, or HIV, or the acuity of their grief, or of what used to be.

This inability to escape mental reminders of a trauma is one of the symptoms of post-traumatic stress disorder (PTSD). Traumatized individuals often experience a "cycle of intrusion and denial" in their continuing efforts to recover from the trauma.[3] At times they are bombarded with "intrusive thoughts"—painful fragments of the trauma that intrude, unwanted, into regular consciousness. Yet other times they may feel numb or disconnected, as if their hardship happened not to them but somebody else.

We all need some respite or escape from reality when the world around us is too grim—a theme at the heart of Manuel Puig's novel *Kiss of the Spiderwoman*.[4] Two men, Valentin and Molina, are incarcerated in a bleak Latin American prison. Valentin, a brave, macho revolutionary, is a political prisoner; the effeminate Molina has been charged with "sex crimes" related to his homosexuality. To maintain his sanity and mentally escape the horror of the situation, Molina spends hours fantasizing, and then narrating to Valentin, intricate old movie plots. He immerses himself in these fantasy creations—comedy, melodrama, camp, romance—to transport himself away from the brutal reality around him. Valentin is annoyed and repulsed: Why must he be subjected to something so trivial? What is the merit of such frivolous nonsense, intruding on the importance of his political beliefs?

Yet as Valentin's imprisonment becomes ever crueler, he, too, comes to welcome these fantasy escapes. They are the only respite available from the horror of his life. He learns the value of creative, reality-bending, denial.

Men who fit the style of Rupture often lack Molina's adaptive ability to transport himself. These are men who are continually bombarded by shards of AIDS—harsh slivers of memory, current jabs of reality, intrusive images of the future. AIDS is always there. How exhausting and maddening this may be—not to be able to escape, to forget, to pretend. What a traumatizing experience in itself, to find no distance from your pain.

Depression

Depression and anxiety are unavoidable and understandable reactions to living with HIV. Some men are able to keep these reactions to a minimum, or develop strategies to manage or counterbalance them. Depression is not the continual backdrop against which they live, not the daily norm.

But men who respond to HIV with a style of Rupture are apt to show some or all the symptoms of a clinical depression. This depression can hinder social relationships or occupational functioning. It can lead to feeling aimless, depleted, hopeless. It can express itself in tears or fury. During the interviews, Ron and Victor described "neurovegetative" signs of depression, such as disturbed patterns of eating and sleeping. Charles' recent bereavement was etched into his face: His countenance and soft voice conveyed his pain as much as his words.

Only Howard seemed to have mastered, or masked, his depression. His style through most of the interview, and I gather in daily life as well, was to be in firm control. He spoke in a tone suggesting a strong command over inner pain. Yet stark emotion broke through at several moments in our interview—brief, fierce storms that suddenly emerged, as if out of nowhere. In those moments, Howard revealed the depths of his usually suppressed despair and rage.

For example, early in the interview Howard smiled as he talked nostalgically, playfully, about the five men in his life who had been his "all-time" favorite sexual partners. Later, however, he began sobbing when they came to mind again. He told me, bitterly: "Do you remember those five guys I told you about? They're all dead."

Similarly, as already mentioned, Howard saw himself as isolated from others. Yet with words quoted at the beginning of this chapter, he did have an ability to connect with others—but only through a bond of desolation and bewilderment. After he mentioned the deaths of these men, he went on:

> It's unbelievable to me that all these young men are dead or dying. . . . I don't understand. There's so little time to do anything, so little that can be counted on. . . . It makes me astonished by how much suffering is in the world. There is so much pain going on, and my exposure to AIDS and people dying somehow makes it all more real to me.

Depression and meaninglessness often go hand-in-hand—people who are depressed often find little meaning in life. One can lead to the other. But they are not the same. Depression has specific symptoms (and can often be treated, with psychotherapy or medication). Meaninglessness is broader—both more encompassing and more diffuse. Depression has at its heart an acute sense of loss; meaninglessness speaks more to emptiness, purposelessness, and disillusionment. An underlying question of severe depression is "How can I live in such pain?" With severe meaninglessness, the question instead is, "Why bother living—what's the point?"

In both situations, men whose life's meaning has been shattered by HIV are at risk for suicide. It can take great courage to continue living amid immeasurable loss and the prospects of a bleak future. Yet suicide in the context of relatively good health (even with HIV) cannot be considered "rational"—it is more likely an expression of hopelessness and interpersonal isolation. By maintaining hope, much that has been ruptured can perhaps be pieced together again. Lives that have been shattered can be reassembled—if not to what they were before, at least to the extent that they no longer lie in broken pieces.

A Process of "Shutting Down"

For some men, HIV prematurely leads to a process of "shutting down" in life. Bob Dylan's words come to mind: "He not busy being born is busy dying."[5] Spiritually, psychologically, emotionally, HIV leads some men to start dying, perhaps long before their T-cells have much impact in the matter. They tend to restrict new activities, initiate few (or no) new adventures, become less accomplishment oriented. Rather than expand their social world, or deepen the intimate relationships they already have, they lean more toward withdrawing and closing themselves off.

Victor and Ron's words, already quoted, echo this sentiment:

Victor: I don't know if I really want to get old. There's not a lot of people left in my life, and I'm worn out trying to make new friends, have them get sick and die. I don't want to be old and alone, I don't know what value there is in surviving for the sake of just surviving. I think, most of the time lately, death might be a welcome relief from what this is, what life has become.

Ron: Ordinarily, at 44 I would not be going through the processes of mourning that I have been, a real sense of closing down that I've experienced in the past several years. This should have been the height of my career, but such as it is, it is.

Many men with HIV experience some aspects of shutting down. But again, men whose primary style is Rupture often lack balance on the other side of the scale—they have no countervailing growth, no compensatory gain. Theirs is not a simultaneous process of expansion and contraction, of growth and grief. Theirs is only the increasing restriction of life and hope.

Recall how Anthony shied away from great career plans: "Career kind of gets to be a joke in some ways. I'm not looking to become the vice president or the president of anything at this point." Yet even with this narrowing, he also put himself through graduate school, got a job, and continued to explore and expand his spirituality. In comparison, Ron's world had also narrowed — but with no concomitant arena of widening. He was withdrawing from his interpersonal contacts, no longer worked, and had no desire or energy to seek out something new. In the same way that his clothes hung too large on his frame, his life, not just his body, was shrinking.

A Pocket of Pride and Personal Defiance

Rupture is rarely complete. To fend off how AIDS may shatter life's meaning, some men strive to isolate and preserve a part of their self-identity as inviolable, as untouched by AIDS. One may be "saturated" in death. AIDS may affect everything—but not this. Even among those men who may be in the greatest pain, one particular, and cherished, aspect of life may shine through their depression and bewilderment.

Invariably, a topic would surface in my interviews with these men that unleashed a surprising torrent of egotism and strength, in sharp contrast to all else that had been said. Like an "AIDS-Free Zone" hidden within the self, this well-protected corner of identity was guarded (and even trumpeted) with defiance and bravado.

For example, Howard's pride in his successful career as an art historian stood in sharp contrast to his sense of irreparable loss and meaninglessness. As the primary realm in his life from which he derived positive self-esteem, his professional stature amply permeated his sense of identity. Howard's ability, and need, to maintain this aspect of his self-view as impregnable to AIDS' impact was revealed by his words:

> A colleague of mine has clearly stated the notion that success comes to those who survive: It's like the second string are now getting to play because the entire first string has died of AIDS. He sees himself as a secondary talent, but one who knows that AIDS will allow lots of people chances that they wouldn't normally get if there weren't these people dying. . . . When I hear that, I tell myself "I'm glad I'm first string." I'd rather die of AIDS than know that I would have been passed over for promotion.

Similarly, when I asked Ron if he ever asked himself "Why me?" he at first responded, simply, that he "happened to be in the right place at the right time." But then he continued, and his demeanor changed. His eyes lit up for the first and only time during our interview, and his voice became infused with a pride that spilled over into piety:

> I've taken part in some of the most incredible of the social experiments of the twentieth century, with great pleasure, and I would say I am totally unrepentant. I've learned a lot.

Victor offered a similar opinion. He regarded his participation in New York's "fast lane" in the 1970s with reverence:

There was a particular thing happening within gay liberation, a sexual kind of freedom, an exploration that was going on that will never, ever, ever happen again. I feel thrilled to have been a part of that and to have witnessed it, because it will never happen again, period.

From one perspective, these quotes, inflated and defiant, could be dismissed as a need to disown a sense of blame, responsibility, or loss. Would Howard *really* prefer to die of AIDS than be "second string?" Do Ron and Victor so relish being part of the gay "social experiment" of the 1970s and 1980s that they would do nothing differently?

But to discredit these words would be a mistake. They may be overblown, but they serve an important function. They represent a part of each man's inner world untouched by AIDS. Such defiance is a stab against meaninglessness, a way to restore purpose to a life plan so brutally derailed. Ron and Victor, as participants in a cutting-edge social movement, and Howard, in his identity as an accomplished academic, hope to unsheathe an adaptive sense of pride as their strongest weapon against the onslaught of meaninglessness that AIDS has unleashed. They cherish these aspects of self-identity in an attempt to salvage a decaying framework of meaning. If they can do so, what a difference that might make.

These, then, are some characteristics of Rupture. These men mourn close deaths, with a grief that feels unquenchable. They cannot distance themselves from AIDS' impact, and so are bombarded with omnipresent reminders of loss. They may be clinically depressed, or suicidal. They have started a process of "shutting down" in their lives. They often identify nothing beneficial that has come from facing HIV—but may hold a strong, perhaps exaggerated pride about one component of their self-identity, in a manner that suggests an attempt to fend off the enormity of their pain.

And many men with this style are angry or rageful. The anger is understandable. It is the flip side of loss, the result of disillusionment, a weapon against inner terror. Contrary to many popular notions, however, I do not see anger as a "stage" that people need to go through. In general, I tend to shy away from stage models of coping because I have not actually seen that people follow predictable stages of facing grief, illness, HIV, or any other major life disruption. Some people may follow these expected patterns, but many do not.

Instead, I see anger more as a pivot in potential growth. Anger often speaks to meaninglessness—but, when harnessed, it can be just as powerful a tool for meaning. Men with a style of Transformation may be no less angry than the men in Rupture, but their anger is harnessed, not diffuse. Angry railing against cruel fate is less productive than angry mobilization against social oppression. The one perpetuates a sense of meaningless; the other can provide purpose.

Again, as with Transformation, I am left to wonder: Why *these* men? Are certain people especially vulnerable to experiencing Rupture? Are there clues in these men's earlier psychological functioning that help explain their sorrow and embitterment in the face of HIV?

With HIV, with other illness and trauma, with growing up in an abusive or alcoholic family—in a host of adverse situations—it is of course true that some people fare better than others. But what leads some of us to do okay and others to crumble?

Some people are quite vulnerable. The slightest disruption of a narrowly ordered life heralds disaster. A minor setback becomes major devastation, the subtlest pressure overwhelms a tenuous capacity to cope with everyday stressors. For these people there are no molehills, only mountains.

Conversely, other people lead lives strewn with the debris of misery. Early losses, tremendous setbacks, unending obstacles — trauma greets them at every turn of the corner. Yet they continually rally or persevere. For them, adversity only strengthens.

And others are a curious combination. Some people weather major crises well, but are oddly unable to negotiate minor stressors. Others display real capability and competence, but only up to a point they dare not cross. Beyond that their resilience collapses and they falter.

Despite much innovative research and theory, there is still much we still do not know about the "why" of how some people fare better than others. Such variability obviously exists—some people *do* fare better, in similar circumstances, from similar backgrounds. More likely than not, it's reasonable to assume that some people may be predisposed to Rupture, based on whatever complicated factors go into coping and resilience. Genes, early childhood experiences, previous struggles with trauma, a capacity for mental flexibility, luck—all these may influence your ability to meet the enormous challenge of forging meaning out of adversity.[6]

Yet there is another side to this coin as well.

Let's look at war. Great attention has been paid to combat-related PTSD, particularly among American soldiers who served in Vietnam. Researchers and therapists have scrupulously examined the lives of men and women who returned from Vietnam, looking for the lingering traumatic effects of war — days, months, and years after military service. Many studies have attempted to answer one of the most crucial of all questions about adversity: Are certain people more likely to develop PTSD?

At first, researchers studying Vietnam veterans assumed that particular individuals would be most prone to the effects of the disorder. Some important criteria would no doubt distinguish those who were most vulnerable—perhaps those with less sophisticated coping mechanisms, or more immature personalities, or from alcoholic families, or with lower IQs.

But this seems not to be the case. Such factors do seem to play a role in the development of a post-traumatic stress reaction—but they are *not* what matters most. In war, far more influential is one's actual degree of combat experience.[7] In Vietnam, the men most likely to develop PTSD were those with the greatest exposure to combat. Witnessing or participating in wartime atrocities had a far greater impact on post-traumatic stress symptoms than any preexisting personality trait. The degree of horror of the situation mattered — the degree to which one's world and selfview were grossly and brutally violated. Not who came from an alcoholic family, what one's IQ was, or how one had previously coped.

The same is likely true with HIV. Long-standing factors of personality or biology are apt to be important in shaping your response to HIV. But they also may be secondary compared to the intensity of loss you experience or the degree of bombardment you face.

If Ron's beloved Robert had not died, would this have buffeted his despair? If Howard forged stronger bonds with other gay black professionals, might this assuage the pain lurking beneath his composed presentation? And I also wonder: Where would Rupture start for me—with how many losses or sorrows, with what particular deaths to mourn, beyond what point of tolerable burden? We all have different thresholds, but we all have *some* threshold. What would it take to cross mine?

In this vein, too, I think back to my friend Robby. A sad irony of his illness and death was that the process had such a transformative effect on all involved except him. We—his caretakers—took away a sense of the paradoxical growth involved in meeting a mortal crisis head-on. Robby appreciated our caring presence and acknowledged understanding our experience, yet did not share in it. His response was certainly one of Rupture.

I wonder: What if Robby had more time to cope and prepare while he was healthy? It was 1984 when he was diagnosed. At 24, Robby did not know he was infected until he was hospitalized with pneumonia. His decline was then steady and relatively swift, lacking even the minor benefit of periods of renewed strength. What if his experience were that of many gay men today—knowing of infection for a long time, years perhaps, while maintaining robust physical health? Would he have been able to gain any advantage if had known earlier? I'd like to think so—yet that, I know, is my own attempt at invoking soothing self-deception to help bring solace.

As I've described them, Transformation and Rupture may come across as polar opposites. I draw them as such for the purpose of definition, but most men will not fit into extremes of any style. Many men who fit the style of Rupture continue to function in life, perhaps getting by with a sadness or bewilderment that never goes away but also never finds full voice. Again, I present these styles as general patterns, not exact blueprints. And as with Transformation, men who experience Rupture differ from each other in some major ways: the extent of actual health impairment, their pre-AIDS social connectedness, and the quantity of loss they have experienced.

However, despite their differences, these men share a common thread of fundamental importance: They have found no meaning, other than senseless loss and despair, in AIDS. Their prior framework for life's meaning has been nullified, and no new beliefs have helped restore it.

What of those men who fall in between these two patterns—or those who outwardly wear the garb of Transformation, looking and sounding the part, but whose inner experience is closer to Rupture? Let's turn to a third style of adaptation, Camouflage.

6

Camouflage: The Fine Line of Self-Deception

Some HIV-positive gay men talk about AIDS and HIV in uncompromisingly positive terms. One man, Francis, began our interview by declaring "HIV is my blessing—I thank God he gave me this blessing to help me grow." As he continued to talk, he admitted no doubt to his gratitude, no blemish to the belief that HIV was, for him, something blessed. To hear him rhapsodize on, the bitter seeds of AIDS had blossomed into a desirable bouquet of flowers. These were roses with all their thorns removed.

Listening to Francis, I had to suspect that his words masked as much as they revealed. Could he mean what he said? It sure sounded heartfelt and earnest, but could it be true?

Camouflage is a style of adaptation where hiding—from yourself, from others—is the main feature of facing HIV and AIDS. This needn't be such a bad thing, and, on first blush, this style bears great similarity to Transformation. HIV infection appears to be a growth-oriented life experience. A person can readily identify positive aspects of living with the virus. He may emphasize these benefits as central to his coping, and may have significant evidence to reflect these gains.

Yet the two styles differ. Among the men I spoke with, I thought that some had actually integrated knowledge of their HIV infection into a new framework for meaning, whereas others had superficially mastered a language of personal growth. Their words glistened with the shiny veneer of change, but other indications suggested the insubstantiality—and potential danger—of this self-proclaimed growth.

Camouflage may do a good job of keeping up a person's spirits. Yet it may actually interfere with effective coping in the long run. The potential danger of this style is that it provides a facade of meaning, not a solid foundation. As such, it may wither or crumble when most needed—in times of crisis such as failing health, when a friend or lover's health worsens, or bereavement. This style of adaptation is like a tree that has lovely branches and glossy leaves, but an inadequate root system. On a calm summer day it looks great, but it can easily topple over when the wind begins to gust.

Let's look at two men whose lives reflect this style, Willy and Francis.

Willy: "You pick yourself up, dust yourself off, and go on"

Willy was a pleasant, extremely polite 34-year-old man whose physical presence suggested more difficulties with his health than he admitted. He looked a bit thin and gaunt. When I arrived for our scheduled, early afternoon appointment, I interrupted an impromptu nap. In addition to AZT and various other prophylactic treatments, Willy was also taking antidepressant medication, and had been since his positive diagnosis two years before.

Willy arranged for our interview to take place at his home. Located on one of Boston's most posh and exclusive avenues, the place I arrived at was magnificent—elegant, stately, baronial. Dark wood, exquisite Oriental rugs, superb antiques, ethereal light filtered through stained glass windows, and there was even a suit of armor on the landing of the stairs. I'd never seen a home quite so museum-like. I felt as if I'd entered Wayne Manor, Batman's (and Bruce Wayne's) palatial estate.

As I was to find out, in some ways it was like Batman's home—only in reverse. Well into the interview, after Willy and I had established a warm rapport, he informed me that this was not, in fact, his place. He lived in the basement, in a separate apartment with a separate entrance. He had a close relationship with his landlord and landlady, who were often away. We were meeting in their living room.

Later, during a break, Willy asked if I wanted to see his apartment, and we went downstairs. It was a tiny, pleasant, spartan affair—well-kept and clean, but lacking all the spectacular grandeur of above.

More than any words spoken during the interview, I think this symbolic confusion of homes, of identities, revealed something essential about Willy's sense of himself in the world. He had wanted me to think of the home upstairs as his—*he* wanted to think of it as his. (He responded to my initial compliments about the house with a gracious and deceptive "Thank you.")

As I later mulled over Willy and our meeting, this incident became the key to understanding Willy's style of coping with HIV. Willy needed to see things other than they really were. This style echoed throughout our interview, like variations on a melodic theme. He inhabited, psychologically and almost literally (at least when his landlord was away), a castle in the sky.

In fact, Willy struck me as a lonely, sad man who was trying, with admirable effort, to put the best face on an overwhelming and deeply frightening situation. He had never had a romantic relationship. His closest friend, George, had died from AIDS-related causes several months before. He lived by himself, with few social contacts and little family. He had spent his adult life working as a waiter at an elegant hotel restaurant, but had needed to stop working earlier that year.

Throughout our interview, Willy had a style of voicing emotionally strong or provocative statements, then quickly recanting or contradicting them. He seemed always to be pulling back. He strained to look for—and perhaps found—the silver lining of whatever potentially negative situation he mentioned. I think he did this in the hopes of stabilizing his world; he needed to keep to an undeviating middle ground, to avoid giving in to any strong emotion.

This style was evident in how Willy described his grief after George's death, as if he needed to catch himself before getting carried away:

> I miss him terribly even now. We used to do a lot together. We were both big fans of antique shows, and canvassing antique shops. We were both avid seashore goers in the summertime, and we used to go to Provincetown quite a bit together. I haven't been to Provincetown since he was diagnosed because he couldn't go, and I didn't feel that my heart was in it. But I've made tentative plans to go there this summer, because he's gone now, and life goes on. After the initial sadness and getting through the funeral and all that, you pick yourself up, dust yourself off, and go on.

Similarly, Willy made several allusions to AIDS as punishment for promiscuity. But he did so only indirectly, and with disclaimers. Willy estimated that from the mid-1970s, when he came out, until the mid-1980s he probably had an average of three or so sexual "trysts" a week. He sometimes met his partners at bars and bathhouses, but more typically in anonymous cruising areas. He maintained this activity for many years, suggesting it was, at least in part, a chosen, pleasurable lifestyle. Yet here, too, he pulls back in his current reflections on that era:

> When I came out, back in 1976 or whenever, my contemporaries were of the feeling that gay men had been so repressed for so long, that, since Stonewall, this was a time to be totally open about your sexuality and as promiscuous as you want to be. I embraced that, but only reluctantly. I say reluctantly because there was something about it that didn't feel quite right. Having sex anonymously in bushes, in bathhouses and things—there was something wrong with it, it didn't feel right to me. I remember even at one point thinking: What could this be doing to your immune system, to be exposed to so many different people all the time in such an intimate way? It must be taxing to your immune system.

These may be accurate remembrances on Willy's part. He may have participated in a cultural and sexual way of life with which he felt incompatible. However, the unusual specificity of his concerns about his immune system, coupled with the length of time he "reluctantly" maintained the activity, suggest that he is retrospectively condemning a sexual style that was, if not ideally suited to him, at least previously acceptable.

Willy's need to protect himself from strong emotion was also evident in his assessment of how other people reacted to his situation. He believed that others felt sadness or anger related to his being gay or HIV-positive, but he did not. For example, Willy told me that he had no difficulty accepting his identity as a gay man. He was "completely comfortable" with his homosexuality. But he added a moment later:

> I've been very fortunate in that everyone I've told about being gay is completely accepting. Now that they know I'm HIV-positive, I get the feeling that they wish it wasn't so, that I wasn't gay. Because if I

wasn't, I wouldn't be HIV-positive. But they've never said anything like that.

And again, when talking about having told his family about his HIV status:

For the most part, it's been a productive thing. I'm glad I did it, they're glad I did it, except for my mother. She's dealing with it as best she can, but she could benefit from talking with someone about it, ideally a group of other parents that are going through the same thing. . . . I think she feels very confused, very helpless and inadequate. She's just consumed with sadness over this.

Willy's words suggest he is using the defense mechanism "projection." With this defense mechanism, a person attributes anxiety-provoking thoughts or emotions to other people rather than acknowledge them within himself. Certainly, Willy's mother may be consumed with sadness. A parents' support group may be of great benefit to her. And people close to him may wish he wasn't gay, because then he likely wouldn't have become infected.

But I suspect that Willy was also consumed with sadness himself, that he also needed support, and that he also ruminated about how being gay (and his particular sexual lifestyle) related to his HIV infection. Yet Willy couldn't allow these disturbing issues into his consciousness. His coping style was to block out unwanted emotion, or project it onto others. He didn't ask himself too many questions, for fear of how unsettling the answers might be.

Willy told me he participated in our interview largely because he was eager to share with me the meaning he found in his HIV infection. In fact, well into the interview (and significantly, not until after he took me to his actual apartment downstairs), he declared that he had been eager to tell me one key piece of information. He then put forth his self-tailored beliefs in reincarnation and "karma." Every soul journeys through various lifetimes, he believed, each time with a distinct lesson to learn. He was quite sure he would live on again after death, in the next step of his karmic ladder.

Willy was certain that his HIV infection had a very specific and literal meaning. His lesson for this lifetime related directly to his infection:

Perhaps in my last lifetime I was a doctor, and the task for me in this lifetime is to learn what it means to be a patient.

These karmic beliefs also assuaged Willy's grief for George. He assumed they would meet again:

Another part of my beliefs about this is I don't think we're just thrown into this willy-nilly. There's a reason why we have relationships with people, and I think our relationships are consistent from one lifetime to another. In other words, George might not be one of my best friends in the next lifetime, but he will be somehow involved in my life in the next life. That made it easier to deal with saying goodbye to him.

With its promises of immortality, reunion, and meaning, Willy said his beliefs in karma calmed him. They made his lot much more bearable. And I believe they did: In the moments of our interview when he elaborated on these convictions his voice changed, as if letting me in on a cherished secret. I doubt it was coincidence that he chose to reveal these things only after our break, after seeing his real home.

These beliefs in karma and reincarnation were crucial to how Willy made sense of his HIV infection, the cornerstone of how he coped. They gave his life, and his foreseeable death, purpose and explanation.

Yet to preserve these beliefs, Willy made a striking contrast between his HIV infection and AIDS in general. This became apparent when, later on, I asked how he made sense of AIDS in the gay community. Suddenly, the laws of karma no longer existed:

AIDS doesn't make sense to me at all. If anything, it's the most unbelievably nonsensible thing I can ever imagine happening. How long have gay men and women been struggling, and we were just starting to accept ourselves, just starting to get other people to accept us, just starting to have a good time, and then this. If anything, it's the worst possible scenario.

And again, when talking about AIDS in general:

I don't think there is a reason why. . . . I don't think there's any answer. It's not a question I waste too much time thinking about.

Willy did not recognize the contradiction in believing that karma existed for him but not for others. To maintain some framework of meaning, he excluded crucial pieces of inconsistent information. Unaware of this discrepancy, distancing himself from what seemed like an underlying belief in punishment, and projecting his anger and sadness onto others, Willy's adaptation to HIV seemed precariously pieced together.

Willy described himself to me as a very orderly person—always making lists, leaving little to chance, sticking to a regular schedule. He disliked disarray. In pragmatic terms, this helped in coping with his HIV: He had written a will, organized his medical care, kept his paperwork in order.

This same style, for better or worse, extended to his emotional world as well. He needed to keep things neat—no strong emotions, no entertaining difficult questions, no loose ends, no admitting the possibility of chaos, randomness, or meaningless into the scheme of his life. His reliance on reincarnation and karma soothed him, bestowing the sense of orderliness he needed.

Yet at some intuitive level, I think Willy knew not to challenge these beliefs too deeply. If he did, he would need to confront a deeper fear, displaced onto others, that "AIDS doesn't make sense to me at all." It is as if Willy wore glasses that give a person crystal clear vision, but only for a very narrow scope. Were he to look farther, or deeper, or from a different angle, everything would become a horrible blur.

Francis: "HIV is my blessing"

I also met with Francis in his home, a visit as revealing and informative as Willy's. A tiny, cramped, colorfully idiosyncratic studio apartment, it was one of those living spaces that seems steeped in the owner's personality. The room struck me as an odd hybrid—part monk's retreat, part little boy's nursery. Along with a cot that functioned as both bed and couch, the place was stuffed with religious relics, Christian statuary, candles, crucifixes, incense, and a tabletop altar. The remaining space was jammed with childhood paraphernalia—shiny pinwheels, campy knick-knacks, toys, and two bright red wagons overflowing with teddy bears. A few piles of spiritual books on AIDS and alcohol recovery were also prominent—interspersed with a slew of humpy beefcake magazines.

Francis learned he was HIV-positive when he was 38, five years before we met. Since then, he had made some dramatic changes in his life. He quit drinking with the help of AA, left an emotionally abusive relationship of many years, and rediscovered the primacy of Roman Catholicism in his worldview. Prayer and meditation had become daily rituals. He had adopted a much more sedate social and sexual lifestyle. Until not long before, his life had been one of pleasurable (and not so pleasurable) indulgence: "Men's fraternities, leather clubs, the Mineshaft, orgies, drugs, the larger the better, the more the merrier . . . I was never satisfied."

Francis was the only study participant who spoke of being whole-heartedly grateful about his infection: "HIV is my blessing. I thank God he gave me this blessing to help me grow." Without the dual stabilizing forces of HIV and sobriety, he believes he would already have died from his alcohol abuse, which he characterized as severe enough to be "life threatening." No longer drinking or drugging, free from his long, abusive relationship, sexually calmer, and actively involved in a spiritual community of seropositive men and women, Francis was living a much healthier life than ever before. His self-esteem had improved. His interpersonal relationships were more fulfilling. He reported that life was both more enjoyable and more meaningful.

These were impressive changes: Here was a man who had come far in a short time. Yet as we continued talking, I sensed just how precarious this growth was. Francis held strong beliefs about personal control, order, and justice—ideas that are not alarming or maladaptive in themselves. But he maintained these views with an unyielding rigidity, leading to ample distortions of reality, in terms of how he viewed others and in how much he hid from himself. The more Francis spoke, the more he seemed to resemble that impressive but dangerously rootless tree.

Francis elicited stronger reactions in me than any of the other men I met with. I came away from our interview feeling overwhelmed—as packed with stimulation as his overstuffed apartment. I admired his pluck. I worried about him. And truth be told, he was the only man I interviewed who made me angry, particularly in the offhand way in which he judged and condemned others.

Believing in personal control was central to how Francis maintained life's meaning in the face of HIV. He repeated, several times and in several ways, "My life is in my hands, I'm responsible for it." This control included believing that people have the ability to forestall, escape, or outwit AIDS:

> I've seen too many people who, when they were diagnosed with the disease, die within a year or six months after being diagnosed because basically they didn't fight it, or because they denied the situation.

Yet after making this statement, and others similar to it, Francis just as frequently repudiated any sense of control: "I think everything is destined to happen when it's going to happen, no matter what." "The ultimate decision is in God's hands." "God's got the game plan, it's his decision where I go and what happens." He also took comfort in the same "denial" that he dismissed in others:

> You can't dwell on it. . . . I take care of myself with the knowledge that I'm trying to keep my immune system together. If I worry about it, I'm going to make myself sick, and I'm going to destroy all the good stuff that I'm doing.
>
> As long as I can learn to read the signs as to what I'm doing with my body, and follow the intuitive hunches as to what to do next, like the diet and the body work, I think I can keep myself together.
>
> I don't bombard myself 100% with [AIDS information], because it gets to a point where enough's enough . . . if I hear or see something of interest, then I will dwell [on] it, but I can't see bombarding myself to the point where I drive myself completely crazy.

With these back-and-forth opinions regarding control, Francis seemed to be accepting responsibility for staying healthy ("My life is in my hands"), but disclaiming responsibility in the event of his own illness ("[It's] in God's hands"). In limited measure, this is a sound strategy—one of the "positive illusions" that help guide us through life.[1] Overestimating a potential for success and minimizing the chance of failure enhances self-esteem and helps keep hope alive.

But with Francis, this strategy seemed to lose its balance. It spilled over into the interpersonal sphere. He held others to a very different standard: *They* died either because "they didn't fight it or because they denied the situation." Death was in God's hands for him, but not for others.

More surprisingly, these beliefs in personal control also led Francis into the sensitive terrain of ranking AIDS' "most innocent" victims:

> The part that really hurts me is the kids: I don't understand kids having the disease. I feel a lot more compassion, a lot more sorrow for them because being an adult, we made our decisions to do what we did, and by making our decisions to do what we did, we allowed ourselves to be open to this virus. Kids to me, what decision did they have? They're born into the world, and because their parents

were drug users, or because their mothers were prostitutes or had slept with a bisexual man, they get infected, they come into the world with this virus. What decision did they make?

Recall that ranking the "guilt" or "innocence" of people with HIV— determining how heartily to "blame the victim"—stems directly from our beliefs in justice and control. Such judgment is not uncommon, yet I've met no other HIV-infected gay man who addressed it so bluntly. I wondered what led Francis to venture into this territory?

Since he hinged this argument on the role of personal control ("we made our decisions to do what we did . . ."), I asked how he accounted for HIV-positive gay men who became infected without having possibly known they were doing something dangerous.[2] He responded without a pause:

Still, we made our decisions. We've got free choice. We did what we wanted to do—we were all having the sex the way we were, it was like the barn door was open and everybody just did it; everything was free and open and wild, let's do it and make up for lost time, or whatever it was.

In other words, even without possibly being able to know that sex was potentially lethal, people were still responsible for their actions, their lives, and, by extension, their infection.

On the one hand, Francis didn't answer my question. I was somewhat taken aback by his response—and it was here that I could not help feeling angry with him. His belief seemed not only illogical, but dangerous. How could people possibly be responsible—and blameworthy—for that which they could not foresee? Was I speaking with a gay man living with HIV— one who had just told me he felt "blessed" because of it—or with some right-wing homophobe?

But stepping back from my anger, Francis did provide an answer, or actually two. First, he revealed that believing in personal control was crucial to his life's meaning. A faulty or inconsistent framework of meaning is better than no framework at all. Francis *needed* to maintain this belief. Logical somersaults and keeping a checklist of innocence were the price he unconsciously paid to maintain meaning in his life—and probably far better for him than having nothing to believe in.

Second, what Francis really blamed was sex. "The barn door was open": The image of sexuality Francis conjured was that of farm animals rutting. As he continued talking, he fleshed out more of his conviction that AIDS' impact in the gay community resulted from gay men's overemphasis on "pleasure." In other words, HIV was a form of punishment.

> For the longest time, gay men basically considered one thing important, and that was pleasure. I mean pleasure sexually, moneywise, partywise, anything that you could add the word pleasure to. . . . For most gay men, pleasure was the only thing that was important. How they got it, where they got it, and with whom, didn't matter. It was the drugs, the booze, the parties.

He then added, somewhat unconvincingly, given what he had just said:

> But I don't look at AIDS as a condemnation or that we're being condemned by God for the fact that we're homosexuals, I don't think that has anything to do with it.

"What *does* it have to do with?" I asked. His answer:

> There was too much emphasis on pleasure. Spirituality was a taboo word for the longest time. Heaven forbid you say to someone you were going to church on a Sunday morning, people didn't want to hear that. . . . Now, there are a lot of gay men I know now getting into all sorts of spiritualities, which they probably never would have done before. They're getting back to the roots that they should have kept, but they threw aside.

Did Francis's stern judgment about the immoral behavior of gay men include him? No. As he had done earlier with the role of denial, Francis delicately distinguishes himself from other gay men, others living with HIV.

In his words above, Francis makes subtle but significant shifts between "we" and "they," either allying or distancing himself from other gay men. When he affirms that AIDS is not God's retribution, he includes himself, here, in the "we" of homosexuals. Yet as he continues, and homosexuals became a pleasure-oriented, misguided lot who strayed too far from their roots, he no longer includes himself in this group: Gay men have become not "we," but "they."

I suspect that Francis is probably not aware of holding himself to a different standard than others. Yet time and again in our interview, he cast himself as separate from (and, by implication, superior to) other HIV-infected gay men. This allowed him to exonerate himself from the blame inherent in his views of sexuality and control and spare himself from being the recipient of punishment—and thus strengthen his self-esteem and maintain, albeit in a rather brittle way, the growth he has achieved.

I do not mean to minimize Francis's real growth. But how are we to understand his words, which he spoke with heartfelt passion yet which lacked so much consistency from one moment to the next? Why such a dogged emphasis on personal control?

Underneath his self-assured language, and despite his real gains, I suspect that Francis was disguising very deep fears of helplessness, of being out of control. He invoked the false surety of his words like an incantation to magically charm away an inner terror.

To the extent that this works, more power to him. Yet the flip side of feeling superior to others is almost always a feeling of frightening power-lessness. And while his belief system clearly had beneficial components, I couldn't help wondering: What does he have to fall back on? What will happen in times of crisis? What inner structure will support him?

In fact, Francis had done very little to prepare himself for the possibility that the course of HIV may go beyond our ability either to "fight" or "deny." His optimistic outlook allowed him to enjoy life, but he purchased this buoyancy with the notion that he was exempt from AIDS:

> I feel like I'm going to wake up and somebody will say "All of this has been a big joke," or that when I go for my tests every six months, they're going to tell me, "Oh, you're negative!" I really don't think about being sick, I think about taking care of myself. I feel as long as I keep doing what I need to do, everything is going to be okay.

Yet in a style that came to feel like one of his most practiced steps in a dance around inner confrontation, moments later he dismissed the same pattern in others:

I only get mad at some of the ones [other gay men] who don't want to admit to or take in the fact of what's going on, who deny the situation.

Francis's gains in the past few years are undeniable. He is in much better physical and emotional shape than he once was. I share his conviction that his life is now richer, his self-esteem stronger. But in some fundamental ways, how Francis ascribes meaning to life has not changed. He has substituted one set of rigid beliefs for another. Francis used to live a life of extreme indulgence; he now lives one of extreme spiritual devotion and sexual condemnation. His incapacity to tolerate ambiguity or anxiety was once disguised with alcohol; it is now disguised (certainly more adaptively, but still disguised) in glib and reactive beliefs about personal responsibility. Instead of facilitating painful self-exploration, Francis's adopted framework of meaning has short-circuited it.

Perhaps Francis exemplifies what psychiatrist Paul Fleischman intended in his book *The Healing Spirit* when he wrote:

The need for a worldview can deteriorate into urgent believing. The hunger for coherence, coupled with the soothing sense of harmony its presence can produce, may turn a worldview into an idol: a static, frozen imitation of reality that is clung to for comfort and security. Religions rush in to cater to this addiction.[3]

In presenting "Camouflage—The Fine Line of Self-Deception," I walk a fine line myself. Why plot this out as a distinct category—doesn't everybody engage in self-deception?

Yes, of course. Self-deception is a basic part of everyday life. Illusions help provide the structure and meaning we need to get by. As we saw in Transformation, benevolently self-deceptive illusions are instumental in getting on with life amid HIV and AIDS. How much better to be able to invoke illusions than not to have them.

Yet illusion must also be tempered with reality. Men with a style of Camouflage have a framework for life's meaning based more on excluding unwanted truths than on confronting them. They may have found helpful ways to compensate and function, but are fending off enormous demons: dread about death and dying. Feelings of inadequacy, powerlessness and helplessness. A profound, hidden fear—perhaps glimpsed consciously, perhaps not—of life as meaningless. And often, the belief that they are to blame for their illness.

The greatest benefit of Camouflage is that it offers protection against the despair of Rupture—a valuable feat when faced with the potentially devastating truths that AIDS and HIV may deliver. But because so much is being kept hidden or disguised, it lacks the flexibility, openness, and potential for deep growth of Transformation.

Camouflage has elements of both Transformation and Rupture, and might best be seen on a continuum with the two. It includes some men who, when you scratch the surface, have a very fragile interior, but also some who are in a process of more substantial growth. Of the four styles, it is the most elusive and difficult to pin down. It is not easily captured in isolated words — many of Francis or Willy's statements, by themselves, sound like those of men I described in Transformation. It is once a variant of Transformation (Francis *did* grow, despite his rigidity) and a truly distinct category (despite their growth, Willy and Francis differed from Anthony and Kyle). It blurs into Transformation and Rupture and overlaps with them, but it's not the same.

Camouflage can sometimes be an important way station on the road to more thorough and substantial change. In this regard, it is like an exaggeration, a caricature of real growth—but one that may become more solid with time.

Imagine a terrified child, alone at night. He repeats to himself over and over, "I am not afraid of the dark, I am not afraid of the dark." These words may be of no help at all, a useless attempt to quell a fear too powerful to conquer. But, on the other hand, they *may* help. By saying them over and over, and listening or reaching for something new as he says them, they may give him a newfound ability to master his fears.

Similarly, some men with this style talk in an extreme, insistent, overly self-confident tone. This reflects their need to block out all threats to a fragile belief system. It's speaking loudly in order not to hear. A person's words—to others, to himself—are unduly amplified, to drone out the terrifying noise of questions that have the power to decimate.

But, like that frightened child struggling in the dark, we can sometimes grow to find substance and meaning in previously empty words. In other words, if the lush but fragile tree of Camouflage can hold on long enough, the roots may indeed find sturdy soil.

Because it is purchased at the expense of true inner scrutiny, this style can be harmful in the long run. It's buying short-term gain at the expense of long-term solidity. With a house built on an inadequate foundation, what, ultimately, will hold the walls up?

Just as harmful, this style can be a destructive tool of social castigation. This is especially true when the need for meaning spills over into blame and self-righteousness. Men with this style, more so than the others, may believe they have a monopoly on the "truth." *Theirs* is the right way of feeling, responding, believing. They have seen the light. We saw this with Francis: his personal growth had become inseparable from judgment, blame, and a harsh ranking of "innocence" among those infected.

How can we characterize Camouflage and distinguish it from the other styles?

Narrower Coping Repertoire

Men with this style tend to have a more limited and less flexible coping style than those I described in Transformation.

Transformation is grounded in accepting the reality of AIDS or your own HIV infection. It acknowledges all the terrible, paradoxical losses that accompany true growth. Camouflage, instead, perches more on denying the psychological reality of AIDS than on coming to terms with very real losses.

For example, compare some of Kyle's beliefs to those of Francis. In some ways these men were quite similar: Both had experienced growth, both had redirected their life as a response to HIV, both seemed on the surface to be doing well. Yet what underlay the changes they had experienced?

For Kyle, it was acknowledging his situation. Although he valued, and often used, his "creative denial," this seemed not to diminish his basic acceptance of reality. Again, his words:

> I know that I'm not getting away from this. It's real, it's here, inside, and how I choose to deal with it is key. . . . I've never had a very strong sense that I could get rid of this, heal myself that way, but I *do* have a strong sense that I can heal myself spiritually and emotionally.

Conversely, Francis's response to AIDS was grounded more in a fantasy of exemption. He admitted the factual reality of his infection, but just as frequently spoke of ways in which he believed he had been (and would be) magically spared, pardoned, or exonerated:

> Sometimes, I feel like I'm going to wake up someday, and somebody will say "All of this has been a big joke," or that when I go for my tests every six months, they're going to tell me, "Oh, you're negative!" . . . I feel as long as I keep doing what I need to do, everything is going to be okay.
>
> I feel sometimes that if I was going to have the virus, or if it was going to be full blown, or something was going to happen, and I should be dead from it, that it would have happened by now.

Notice how Francis does not say the word "AIDS." He uses a more roundabout (and distant) phrase, "if it was going to be full blown." I suspect that he automatically censored himself from saying the words "If I were to get AIDS. . . ." To say them out loud would be too threatening, too close. He avoids them, so as to not jinx himself or invite trouble.

This difference in coping styles relates, in large part, to the type and nature of defense mechanisms each of us uses.[4] We all rely on defense mechanisms to deal effectively with the anxieties, pains, and fears (small and large) that crop up on a regular basis. Defenses are a form of necessary protection, of helpful adaptation to difficult circumstances. It's often a very fine line between what's "defensive" and what's protective—after all, when our defense mechanisms help protect us from unwanted anxiety, this is often of adaptive benefit.

Defense mechanisms are not maladaptive in themselves. They only become a problem when they don't work properly. At the risk of oversimplifying, often this happens when they become too weak or too strong. When too weak, they don't offer adequate protection. A person can't muster appropriate self-insulation against the major tribulations, or minor irritations, of life. Such is the case in Rupture: These men can no longer employ an adequate level of defense against the ravages of their situation.

Conversely, when defenses are too strong, they limit our access to new knowledge, insight, or experience—all of which are necessary for growth. They may block out unwanted anxiety, but they also distort the ability to perceive ourselves and the world honestly and openly.

Think of defenses as protective outer clothing. Common wisdom (and many a mother's advice) suggests that the most effective way to dress in severe weather is with layers of clothing. Particular layers can be donned or shed as the temperature changes. So too with defenses: ideally, there's enough to protect and cover adequately, but not so much as to stifle. And they can be added or withdrawn as the situation warrants.

In Transformation, the layering seems to work right. Those men balance being protected against the elements but not smothered. Alternatively, for those men in Rupture, defenses are threadbare and tattered—a bone-chilling cold blows right in. Daily existence is like life in a severe clime with inadequate means for warmth.

In Camouflage a person may have protection, but not in layers. The protection comes more in the form of a large cumbersome coat that always needs to stay on. Without it, you are helplessly exposed. It may help block out the cold, but it offers no flexibility. It's either on or off, and it dare not be shed—for underneath, perhaps no other protection is available.

Francis's growth was grounded in the exclusion of unwanted truths, Kyle's on their examination. Kyle's defenses, including denial, seemed to work in layers that offered some degree of flexibility. For Francis, it was more "all or nothing."

In this regard, Camouflage calls to mind the Greek myth of Procrustes and his infamous bed. Procrustes (caring soul that he was) regularly offered lodging to weary, unsuspecting travelers. He had a special iron bed just for this purpose. How hospitable of him—except that people had to fit the bed exactly. And being made of inflexible iron, the bed had one size only. Procrustes's guests, therefore, were either decapitated or stretched to fit accordingly.

For men with this style of adaptation, their defensive structure—and how this influences life's meaning—is like a Procrustean bed. Facts are distorted to accommodate the inflexibility of the framework. It's one size fits all; the bed (framework) doesn't change. Information and emotions that are incompatible are thrown out, altered, or ignored.

On the surface, this often gives rise to inconsistencies in a person's presentation. What is proclaimed one moment may be disavowed the next. What sounds like a heartfelt revelation is soon forgotten or supplanted with an equally heartfelt, and incompatible, revelation.

We see this with both Francis and Willy. Francis describes his pre-HIV days as quite hedonistic. His life revolved around revelry: "Men's fraternities, leather clubs, the Mineshaft, orgies, drugs, the larger the better, the more the merrier . . . I was never satisfied." Later, however, as he condemns this same lifestyle because it placed "too much emphasis on pleasure," he talks as if he had never participated in it.

Of course, inconsistency is part of the human condition. We are all too multifaceted to be devoid of contradictions. But here, I speak of a sense of abrupt discontinuities from one moment to the next, in terms of what people believe or how they see themselves.

In psychotherapy, I sometimes present my patients with a metaphor of still photographs versus motion pictures. Some people live as if life were a series of still photos. They act as if what they feel and think in that moment is the entire picture, with no connection with what has come before or what might follow. They forget that they have felt or acted or thought differently. Yet motion pictures are more accurate—who we are, and how we engage in life, are captured more in an unceasing flow of continuity and change than in an isolated moment.

The inconsistencies of men with this style are like disconnected still photos. This differs from paradox, where the essential unity of opposites is acknowledged, even if the contradictions do not occur in the same moment.

"HIV as Punishment"

The representation "HIV as Punishment" is another main underpinning of Camouflage. For many men, the hidden belief "I am to blame for my illness" is one of the major impediments to deeper growth.

Believing in punishment resides more between someone's words than in explicit statements—it is found in judgment of gay hedonism, or condemnation of other gay men, or in displaced or projected feelings of shame or guilt onto others. Willy and Francis both seem to hold a disowned belief in punishment. Francis talked disparagingly about gay men's "emphasis on pleasure." Willy "reluctantly" participated in the anonymous cruising he saw as "wrong." Neither explicitly said that AIDS was punishment, but both nonetheless seemed to believe this was the case.

"HIV as Punishment" is not absent among men with other styles of adaptation. However, nowhere else is it as prominent—or as noisily disclaimed. Denying a hidden belief in punishment occupies a great deal of

Francis and Willy's psychic energy; they invest a great amount in not allowing themselves to feel blamed.

The Denial of Grief

Men with this style may not be able to admit to themselves the enormity of their grief. Those described in Transformation have worked through many of their losses; those in Rupture are overwhelmed by them. In contrast, Camouflage often has, at its base, a fear that grief would be intolerable, beyond one's capacity to bear. As such, grief is not just put aside. It is shunted out of awareness.

This question—what can be faced, what is intolerable—is a struggle that all of us subtly renegotiate throughout life. This is particularly true in times of crisis. One of the great benefits of psychotherapy is that it may broaden and strengthen a person's tolerance — for feared or disquieting emotion, for loss, for anxiety, for disliked parts of ourselves, for expanding our vision beyond the moment, for disappointment, for the ambiguities and uncertainties of life.

People vary dramatically not only in their real ability for tolerating these things, but also in their *assessment* of what they can tolerate. The assessment does not always match the fact. In other words, many of us routinely underestimate or overestimate our ability to tolerate stress, internal or imposed from without.

Despite a potential outward show to the contrary, some men tend to fear that admitting the reality of their situation would be intolerable — the accompanying grief would be too much to bear. To admit such cataclysm, to open themselves up to that pain, would be to risk devastating consequences.

What are the consequences people most commonly fear? Perhaps it is a fear of going crazy, of having a "breakdown." Perhaps it's the fear of loss of control (this was the case, I think, with Willy, and how he always reined in emotions whenever they threatened to gallop, or even broke into a trot). Perhaps it's a fear of suicide, that you could not tolerate that much psychic pain without killing yourself. Perhaps it's the fear of crying. Or the fear that you might start crying and never be able to stop.

In contrast with men with a style of Transformation, in Camouflage, a person assumes that grief would be intolerable. Yet I suspect that despite this self-assessment, these men vary in their actual capacity. For some, the fear of admitting pain or grief can be nudged and nurtured into a deeper capacity for tolerance. The fear is more the impediment than the fact.

For others, however, the fear may be well founded. Perhaps some of us do *not* have the capacity to bear. Emotion too intense, questions too disruptive, pain too deep—all of these might in fact destroy a growth tenuously perched on half-truths. Not all people are created equal, or develop equally. We diverge greatly in how much anxiety and trauma we can manage.

So for some men, Camouflage is a marvelous accomplishment, growth beyond any previous expectations. For others, it is merely a resting point. They will learn, in time or with additional experiences, that they have the requisite strength for more arduous journeys.

In either case, the men who reflect this style are often those who prevent themselves from grieving the profound real losses that AIDS and HIV entail. Perhaps they don't need to grieve, or can't, or shouldn't. Camouflage may be the most adaptive response, given a person's capacities — but it likely caps the possibility of more substantial change.

Separating Individuals from Community

Finally, men with this style of adaptation develop subtle but prominent strategies to differentiate between themselves and others.

With Francis, we saw this repeatedly. It was a main feature of his self-presentation. AIDS afflicted other gay men because of hedonism, but for him it was a "blessing." Others died because either "they didn't fight it . . . or . . . denied the situation," but his choice was not to "dwell on it."

Willy did the same thing, less pervasively but to the same end. An individual belief in karma provided him with a sense of purpose so soothing and pleasant that he snuggled into it like a comfortable afghan. He wrapped himself in his beliefs for warmth and assurance. But the same virus, in other men, "made no sense at all."

In distinguishing yourself from others, in splitting between your own HIV and AIDS in general, what is overlooked is the dreadful massiveness, the nonsingularity, the nonindividuality, of AIDS' impact. Someone may resurrect meaning in the context of his own life—but how to explain the terrible fact that so many lives, so many communities, are grappling with the same devastation?

Could Willy sustain the belief that if it's karma for him, then it's also karma for everyone else? (Could *everybody* have been a doctor in a former lifetime?) Could Francis allow that if others are paying the price of hedonism, then he is as well? That others may be exactly like him—frightened, pained, readjusting to an unwanted and unforeseen fate?

These thoughts are the rational extension of how Willy and Francis create meaning in their lives. Yet to admit the logic of them would jeopardize the growth they had achieved. They lop off a central fact about AIDS—its enormity—to render it more manageable. This helps provide meaning and structure, but it ignores the heart of AIDS' most devastating feature.

This differs from the men I discussed in Transformation. For them, a central theme was their sense of belonging with other gay men, or others with HIV. It is *we* who are infected, who are affected. An "us" is involved. Kinship becomes a springboard for meaning. With Camouflage, the communal tragedy of AIDS is not acknowledged. It may even need to be kept out of mind. It is *me* who is infected—I'm different from the others.

Much of the spiritual and inspirational literature on AIDS, and the glib personal growth movement that seems to wax and wane around the epidemic, draw men with a style of Camouflage. A mass of people who face a life-threatening crisis make for willing recruits (and consumers). The hunger for meaning can be extraordinarily compelling. Any system of beliefs that can seduce with the false promise of easy meaning will find avid followers, especially among people facing tribulations such as AIDS.

This is not to say, of course, that HIV cannot trigger true and remarkable change, spiritual or otherwise. It can, and does. But it is often the craving for meaning that draws people, rather than the true apprehension of it, a facade of purpose more than the fact of it. Spirituality can be a unique entrance into a world where life's meaning is redefined, a world that lacks any comparable gateway. Yet a spiritual journey can just as easily lapse into a "static, frozen imitation of reality that is clung to for comfort and security."[5]

Whatever underlies its motivation, the appeal of Camouflage is understandable, whether expressed in spiritual terms or not. In times of great crisis, a person's central psychological challenge is to maintain or recreate a view of life as meaningful. To meet this end, a facade of meaning may be better than no meaning at all.

I suspect that in contrast to men with other styles, neither Francis nor Willy—nor others similar to them—would want me defining their adaptation in this manner. Francis and Willy felt theirs was true and important growth. Who am I to tell them otherwise?

If given the opportunity, *would* I tell them otherwise? Perhaps, if I felt confident enough in my judgment that they were ready to confront their fears in a more direct way. But just as likely I would say nothing.

Years ago, I learned a crucial lesson about effective psychotherapy from a short story by Carson McCullers, "Madame Zilensky and the King of Finland." On the surface, the story has nothing to do with psychotherapy —yet it has been as instructive as any theory or textbook I have seen.

Madame Zilensky is a lively and eccentric music teacher. Her colorful past, as recounted in her frequent stories, seems too wonderful to be true —and it is. It gradually dawns on a colleague of hers, Mr. Brooks, that most everything Madame Zilensky says is a lie to glamorize herself, including her many tales about a long-standing friendship with the King of Finland.

With prosecutorial relish, Mr. Brooks leads Madame Zilensky into repeating one of her tales about the King and then springs his trap: "Madame Zilensky," he screams out, "there *is* no King of Finland . . . Finland is a democracy!" He is correct, but the glee in his triumph quickly vanishes as he watches her crumble. Too late, Mr. Brooks realizes the foolishness of robbing someone of something so important, even if it is false.

It is far too easy to play Mr. Brooks. Truth runs deeper than mere fact. Being a psychotherapist is sometimes about offering a person truth, but it is just as often about sustaining the illusions that help.

If he were mine and I needed him, I would not want someone taking the King of Finland away from me, lie or not. I hope I offer the same respect to others. We all have our Finnish monarchs. Until a person no longer needs him, long live the King of Finland.

7

Impassivity: Minimizing the Trauma

Jules: I consciously try not to let HIV be this all consuming thing in my life. I don't define myself as an HIV-positive person. A lot of people I've met have almost become professional HIV-positive people. They live that every day of their lives, they're really into it. I don't want to be like that.

Sam: My day-to-day life has not been much affected. . . . I don't detect any real change in who I am as a person, other than maybe opening me up a bit more. . . . I carry on a normal life. If you don't dwell on it, you can do things pretty normally.

Craig: I don't know that I really deal with it. I think it's just kind of there. I don't give it a lot of attention, that's how I deal with it.

*F*or some men, HIV has neither transformed how they understand the world and themselves, nor robbed them of a once-viable framework and left them with nothing. It has not shaken their world to the core. They have not renounced old patterns, changed their relationships, or joined new groups. No hoopla, drama, despair, or conversion-type experience. These men say that HIV has had only minimal impact on their self-concepts or worldview, and the evidence of their lives supports this. For these men, HIV simply seems not to be that big a deal.

In the style of adaptation to HIV I call Impassivity, the profound and earth-shattering fact of HIV infection seems — well, not so profound or earth-shattering. Ron and Victor (described in Rupture) each bemoaned

147

how AIDS had "changed everything." Men with styles of Transformation and Camouflage speak similarly of AIDS' massive impact. In contrast, some men are more apt to believe that AIDS has changed nothing, or only very little. Life is still life, the world is still the world, I am still myself. Their attitude seems to be, more than all else, one of surprising indifference.

Sam and Craig typify this style.

Sam: "If things happen, they happen — that's life"

Sam had just turned 50 a few weeks before we met. He had known he was HIV-positive for five and a half years. He was talkative, frank, and seemingly completely unabashed about revealing personal details of his life. He had a manner about him that was at once gruff and gentle, uneducated but psychologically astute. Despite a low T-cell count (140), Sam's health had not been greatly affected by the virus.[1] Neither had his fundamental beliefs about life, death, or himself.

Sam and his lover, Joseph, lived in a mid-sized, pleasant, rather unkempt suburban home in a working-class neighborhood. They had been together for about four years, since after Sam's positive test result. Joseph had AIDS. Each had children from a former marriage, teenagers and older, who visited occasionally but lived independently or with their mothers. Joseph still worked, despite being ill; Sam had recently gone on disability, reluctantly, at the (dubiously legal) insistence of his employer. He had worked with the same construction firm for 25 years, first as a laborer and then as a foreman.

An important theme in Sam's life, since a few years prior to HIV, was "making up for lost time." When he and his wife divorced 12 years earlier, Sam had "no idea" that he was gay, or bisexual. He traced for me the path by which he had stumbled onto his erotic pleasure in men:

> I was married for 15 years, separated in 1979, had my first gay experience two years after that. I didn't realize I was gay before that. When I had my first experience I was about 40. . . . I had a girlfriend who turned me on to some books on sexuality. These books were separated into straight, bisexual and gay histories, and there were case histories. I found myself being turned on by the descriptions of gay and bi sex. . . . I realized that gay and bi personal ads, which I had read over the years and used to think funny, were

turning me on, I was attracted to them. So I decided to answer one.
I'm surprised that I wasn't nervous, but I wasn't. But I was still shun-
ning the gay part. At that time, I convinced myself that bi would be
okay. . . . the first couple I got involved with, he and I made it
together and I enjoyed it so much that the gay repression went out
the window, to hell with that! So I accepted it almost overnight, and
tried to catch up on what I had been missing.

So in his early forties (in the early 1980s), Sam indeed "tried to catch
up." He loved sex with men. He tricked up to four or five times a week,
"depending on how much time I had." With the enthusiasm of a connois-
seur, he scrutinized and ranked various means of meeting partners: He
favored the personal ads, which he worked "like a pro." He didn't care for
bars, having "never figured out how that scene worked." And although he
didn't go to bathhouses (he maintains he was unaware of their existence),
he did become a regular devotee of private orgies scheduled twice monthly
in someone's home. Most of his encounters were one-night events, but a
few men became regular sex partners. Until he met Joseph, he had neither
an ongoing relationship, nor interest in one.

The same kind of nonchalance that characterized Sam's coming out
in midlife also carried through to learning he was positive, living with HIV,
and dealing with Joseph's AIDS. He registered all of these events with a
distinct nonreaction. His life was barely affected by receiving a positive
test result:

When I found out I was infected, I was kind of down, but not for
long. I can go on and not think about it. I don't deny it to the point
where I don't keep track of myself and get medical help . . . but at
the same time, I can just deny and that doesn't bother me at all. I
think it's a healthy mechanism, because I've run across a lot of other
people that are really out of it, that stay in the dumps for months
and months.

At first after learning he was positive, even Sam's sexual lifestyle remained much the same, although he tried (with mixed results) to pay more
attention to safe sex. Ultimately, what changed Sam's activity was HIV's
effect on the world of gay sex, rather than its effect on him per se. It
became more difficult to meet men. The bi-monthly orgies stopped. A few

of his regular tricks got sick or died. And so when he met Joseph through a personal ad, and Joseph wanted to form a relationship with him, he thought it a convenient and sound idea.

Sam thought that he and Joseph had a difficult relationship:

> I don't think we'd still be together if it weren't for this [HIV]. . . . If the situation were different, I would have ended things, we've had too many disagreements. But it's hard to say—it's not a nice thought to say we're together just because of this, and that wouldn't be entirely accurate, either. But I think some blow-ups would have come along where it would have been easier to say goodbye, whereas now we can't just say goodbye, so we have to make up, so then we're happy again. If we didn't have this to keep us together, it would have been easier to walk out.

In certain ways, HIV has had an important impact on Sam's sense of himself, of how to be in the world. In Chapter 3, I described how Sam saw HIV as a relief and how he used HIV as a strategy for attention.

Sam described himself to me as someone who was "pretty quiet . . . who keeps to himself an awful lot." This seemed accurate: I saw it reflected in his demeanor, his tone of voice, his attitudes about life. He struck me as a rather content, even-keeled man. Not timid, but someone who tended to blend into the woodwork. But how he loved the drama of telling people about his HIV! Yes, he was "pretty quiet"—but quiet men don't usually air their dirtiest laundry with such public delight.

Sam relished disclosing his HIV status and his formerly secret homosexuality. He told his co-workers, his children, his siblings, his ex-wife, his nephews and nieces—it seemed anyone he could think of, or perhaps anyone who would stop and listen. It was the same impetus, I think, that led him to regale me with explicit details of his sexual escapades. There was a quirky exhibitionist lurking inside him, and why hold back now?

The way Sam "enjoyed the drama" of telling people that he was gay and HIV-positive likely had an adaptive benefit. He felt empowered by it. It helped neutralize his own potential sense of guilt or shame. It provided him an ideal conduit to escape his own long-ingrained sense of himself—his quietness, his ordinariness. And I suspect it became a vehicle to constructively channel anger—anger at society, at people who thought they knew him, at being pegged as a certain type of person. (He reminded me of a man I saw in psychotherapy, an exceptionally clean-cut businessman with a racy tattoo on his back. He entertained the frequent fantasy of shocking his co-workers by showing it to them.) Here, at last, was Sam's way to distinguish himself, to seize the spotlight.

Yet despite these growth-oriented changes, Sam's overall adaptation to HIV was overshadowed by a much more pervasive response to his situation. At some deeper level, AIDS seemed inconsequential in how Sam made sense of life, the world, and himself.

HIV's nonimpact on how Sam found meaning in life was summed up in his response to my question, "Do you ever ask yourself 'Why'—why me, why AIDS, why gay men?" Interrupting the easy flow of our conversation, Sam looked up at me as if I had suddenly begun speaking a foreign language. Surely this was not a new thought to him? But he answered, "No, I don't ask that, it's never entered my mind. I don't know why not, but I don't."

He went on to identify the "resignation" that he sees as central to his approach to life:

> One thing I probably picked up from my mother is a resignation to things that happen to you. If things happen, they happen—that's life. It's almost fatalistic. Anything bad that happens, I don't feel too badly about—if I'm poor, I'm poor. That's life. I can very easily adapt, take the attitude "C'est la vie" and not think anymore about it. If I'm lucky, fine, if I'm not lucky, fine, do the best I can—which I guess at this point is a pretty healthy attitude to have.

Throughout the interview, Sam repeatedly reconnoitered back to this main point:

> My day-to-day life has not been much affected, other than a few project-type things.
>
> I don't detect any real change in who I am as a person, except for opening me up more. But I have such a big history of being relatively closed that while it's opened me up more, it's not to the point of making me an open person.
>
> I carry on a normal life. If you don't dwell on it, you can do things pretty normally.

Has HIV changed any of Sam's friendships or relationships?

It probably has, but I can't think of how, or who. I feel closer to other people because I can open up more, but looking at the relationship objectively, removing myself from myself to look at it, I don't see much change. So I'm tempted to say yes, but I don't know how.

Has Sam experienced any benefits or gains from being positive?

No, not much. I guess you take a more serious view of life and what you're doing. Maybe you use your time better, but I don't really—a lot of people say they do that, but I'm not sure they do. . . . Overall, it hasn't change my view too much.

This sense of acceptance, which he labeled "resignation" or "fatalism," seemed to be one of the most salient aspects of Sam's psychological make-up. It did not strike me as simply a mask for deeper feelings, or a defense mechanism such as rationalization. It was thoroughly woven into his descriptions of past events, current turmoils, future concerns. It was also evident in his attitude about his relationship with Joseph. Despite their difficulties, Sam had resigned himself to the idea that they "had" to be together because of HIV: "We can't just say goodbye, so we have to make up."

The nonchalance with which Sam greeted major life events also characterized the process of our interview itself. Understandably, my interviews with all of the men elicited strong, varied reactions. Some cried. Some spoke with a quiet reverence, others with a fierce anger, others with a lovely, wistful humor. Many expressed deep pride in their accomplishments, conveyed in their tone as much as their words.

Sam did none of these things. He spoke matter-of-factly, with an honesty that felt quite genuine. But there were no tears, no awkward pauses, no subtle deflections away from inner fears too frightening to verbalize. In the evenness of his voice and manner, in the casualness of it all, we could have been talking about the weather.

A second theme also seemed central to Sam's psychological makeup, perhaps related to this resignation: Sam did not like uncertainty in his world. He wanted to know what was happening—not only with pragmatic issues, but with larger, amorphous questions as well.

For example, Sam did not see any likelihood of escaping AIDS. He believed the "progression rate [from HIV] is still 100%." He dismissed as unrealistic any hope for a medical breakthrough: "I think it's more likely that they come up with a vaccine rather than a cure." Similarly, he had contemplated the issue of his own death, and decided to his satisfaction questions of an afterlife:

> My mind's pretty much made up that . . . when I'm dead, I'm going to be dead, and that's the end of everything.

Again, given what I had come to expect from the other men I spoke with, I was surprised to hear Sam talk about such profound matters so matter-of-factly. He displayed no horror or relief, no obvious self-deception, no sense of religious calm. He was just matter-of-fact. I asked how it felt to talk and think about these things—angering, sad, confusing?

> No. Of course, I'd just as soon that they would come up with a cure. But again, I can resign myself to the fact that you've only got so much time on this earth. I've got to go sometime anyway.

Perhaps Sam's exhibitionistic quality, his decision to tell everyone about his infection, related to this need to jettison uncertainty from his life. Being so public with HIV removed one of the great sources of ambiguity in all our lives: maintaining a private identity distinct from our public one. As with his belief that AIDS was inevitable, and having "made up" his mind about death's finality, perhaps telling everyone about his HIV was a way for Sam to further prune the untidiness of ambiguity from his world.

In short, HIV seemed not to be a major trauma for Sam. It was unwanted, certainly—but hey, that's life. His infection had led to no great epiphanies, no horrible anguish. He took good medical care of himself and faced the future pragmatically. He did not by any means ignore HIV's presence, but it caused only minimal disruption in his previous understanding of life and the world. Relying on several representations of HIV—Relief, Strategy, and Confirmation of powerlessness—Sam faced his current struggles much as he had previous life challenges: with a shrug of the shoulders, a resignation more benign than embittered, and a general sense that, overall, "I've had a pretty good life."

Craig: "I don't give it a lot of attention"

Craig had a definite talent for words. He approached topic after topic in our interview with a deft cleverness—one bon mot, one quip, one colorful allusion after another. He frequently smiled, flirtatiously and proudly, as punctuation (or self-congratulation?) for his incisive remarks. He told me he had written (but not published) three novels, a screenplay, and some "politically correct pornography." The paralegal work he did to earn money "had nothing to do with" his sense of identity.

Craig was 30 when we met. A positive test result 18 months earlier came as no surprise; it only confirmed what he had long assumed. Craig's first two lovers had both died of AIDS-related causes. His physician had been tracking his declining T-cells for several years. The test itself was simply "gilding the lily."

Being gay had long been central to Craig's self-identity. He came out when he was in high school. Gayness for him meant "much more than just having sex with men"—it was a worldview, a way of life, an elite member-ship in a privileged, ancient culture. Our interview was peppered with refer-ences to Walt Whitman, gay shamans and berdaches in Native American societies, the "spiritual, transcendent" aspects of homosexuality. In response to my opening request that he tell me a little about himself he asserted, "I am a gay person, first and foremost, and that colors the way I look at every-thing."

This sense of gay pride and solidarity was crucial in Craig's response to AIDS. As already stated, Craig saw the disease as meaningless, but gleaned great satisfaction from the gay community's response:

> No, it's senseless, it's just a disease. . . . What there *is* to be made sense of, and to be proud of, is the reaction to it, and to learn from that. On the whole, gay people have responded brilliantly: We've developed support networks, support groups, groups to raise money and dispense caring to people who need it. We've learned how to deal with our own bereavement, on the whole, as a people.

In this regard, Craig's response to HIV was a growth-oriented one. It furthered his already strong sense of gay belonging. But, as with Sam, Craig's more encompassing response to HIV and AIDS was one of indif-ference. Craig, who held a graduate degree in theater and clearly enjoyed the pleasures of juicy wordplay, seemed to be facing the real drama of his life with marked nonchalance.

Craig had an attitude about his infection that was unique among the men I've known with HIV: He refused to take it seriously. It's not only that he used wit to fend off hidden pain and fear, although there was surely some of this at play. It seemed more than that. Despite the travails he had already been through, Craig somehow refused to accept the reality of HIV's power.

Craig's manner reminded me of *la belle indifference*. Until the early twentieth century, one of the most common psychological disorders was hysteria, or what we now refer to as Conversion Disorder. Hysteria involves paralysis of some part of the body, without an adequate physiological explanation. Perhaps someone loses the ability to walk, or talk, or see. Often, people with this disorder display a puzzling nonchalance about their impairment. This marked lack of concern is called *la belle indifference*. Craig was not paralyzed, he had no Conversion Disorder. But his grand indifference was hard to connect with the facts of his life.

Behaviorally, Craig took appropriate prophylactic measures. He practiced safe sex with his current lover, took AZT, and attended adequately to a health regimen of good diet, sleep, and exercise. He knew he had the virus and acted accordingly. But he gave no indication of psychologically acknowledging the potency, reality, or explicit danger posed by HIV. He treated it as a trivial inconvenience, a nuisance he begrudgingly had to tolerate:

> I'm annoyed by HIV, I'm bored by it, I'm fatigued by it. I wish the ring around AZT came in different colors. I wish they had AZT with iron. I want something different. It's a pain in the ass being HIV-positive.

As he continued, his voice conveyed neither dismay nor fear, but simply irritation. He sounded put out, inconvenienced. How else had HIV had an impact on his life? He went on, and he spoke like a child deprived of a too-expensive toy:

> I'd like to be able to go on safari to see the gorillas, and I don't think I'll be able to go there. I can't eat sushi now. Well, I happen to like sushi, and I can't have it. I like smoking pot sometimes, I can't do that. It's these little things, it's a real pain in the ass. . . . It's a nuisance.

Not able to eat sushi? Can't go on safari? In some ways, these were the most provocative and unusual beliefs I heard in any of the interviews.

Irreparable loss, punishment, spiritual trigger: These I expected. Each captures an aspect of facing major trauma. These responses vary tremendously in their content, yet all share undeniable respect for the virus's potential lethality. AIDS may be hated, feared, joked about, railed against, or embraced, but its authority is rarely doubted.

Craig was the only participant who did not accord HIV this stature. Other men also joked about HIV, sometimes with crisp dark humor. (Nate comes to mind here. He quipped, rather drily, "I'm fascinated by the HIV virus, how it attaches to cells, how it works. I thought, 'Well, if I have to be knocked down by something, isn't it nice that it's as clever as this. So chic, so cutting edge.'")

Such joking typically strikes me as a sound means of negotiating the reality of AIDS' impact. But Craig seemed not to respect the virus. He of course knew it was there, but his attitude was such that he wouldn't deign to give it its proper due. He treated HIV with a sense of dismissal, as if it were beneath him. The virus was an uninvited visitor with no letter of introduction. He would not grant it an audience.

This attitude may have struck me as more expectable in someone for whom AIDS remained distant. For some men, an HIV-positive diagnosis lacks substance or tangibility. It is a piece of paper with lab results, a fact laden with portent but short in actual physiological or emotional impact. The person feels and lives the same—no ill health, no weight loss, no sick or dying or dead friends.

But that was far from Craig's situation. His previous lovers had died and so had a close friend. Another friend, his "closest," was also positive, and symptomatic. Craig was taking AZT. Yet despite the nearness of these losses and impingements, his indifference to the reality of HIV was similar to that of some men who have had no contact with AIDS or bereavement:

> I imagine if I got sick it would change things, but until then, I deal with it mostly by not paying much attention to it. . . . I don't feel like I'm going to get sick next week, or next year. I think I'm good probably for another five years before anything bad will happen to me—and five years is far enough away that it doesn't mean anything. I don't have an image of me seriously getting sick.

Later in the interview, Craig decided that even his getting sick would probably not "change things." He again demonstrated the same minimization of HIV's impact that allowed him to call it "a nuisance":

I suppose if I got sick I'd freak out, but so far I haven't gotten sick, so it's not an issue. No, I don't know that I'll freak out: I may be too busy. I imagine that if I got sick—everyone else that got sick, they're too tired to have any emotion about anything, they're just busy, then when they get better, they get a little cranky. I'm good at being cranky, so that shouldn't be a problem.

He concluded with a coda of magical thinking: "Then after that, I guess I'll be all better again."

Craig did not think AIDS had changed him in any significant personal way. It reaffirmed his pride in being gay, but this had been important to him already. Were there any other changes?

No, I don't think it's affected who I am. . . . I'm still who I was, but it puts another spin on it. It's another thing that goes into me that makes me look at the world in a certain way, but it hasn't created any kind of real change.

How did he deal with living with HIV? Again, the same indifference:

I don't know that I deal with it: I think it's just kind of there. I don't give it a lot of attention.

Any benefit, any personal gain, any sense of learning something from the adversity?

It would be a shame if I had to say no, but I don't think so. To some extent, any kind of illness is going to make you more compassionate of other people who are ill with your illness, or with another illness. . . . But by and large, no. It would be like being in an auto accident: Was there anything good about it? No, but it makes you a little bit more aware of the use of safety belts. So, big deal. Now I know to exercise three times a week. I don't think that's a good trade-off.

In short, Craig's jocular, sardonic tone remained consistent throughout the interview. He discussed his lovers' deaths, his own health concerns, his strained relationships with his family, all with the same clever detachment. He communicated a curious blend of cynicism and optimism. Nothing seemed of great value, but he certainly wasn't going to let a small thing like HIV get him down.

Was Craig's attitude "defensive"? Perhaps. As we spoke, I wondered where the pain or fear or rage were. I assumed they lurked in some hidden corner, masked by his witty veneer. I tried a variety of probing questions and styles to get at it. But his response never wavered.

More so than defense, I came to think that Craig simply did not experience HIV as an emotional trauma. AIDS had neither embittered nor mellowed him. It signaled neither collapse nor revitalization. In an odd way, in the scheme of his own life Craig saw HIV as irrelevant. With the exception of a strengthened sense of gay belonging ("I consider gay men and women my people"), AIDS had not affected how Craig made sense of life and the world. It had led to no crisis of meaning.

And in fact, despite his disregard for the reality of what AIDS had already done and could do, he was doing fine. He derived strength and support from his relationship with his current lover, who was HIV-negative. He "tolerated" work, just as he had before. In most every regard, he functioned just as he had previously.

In a rather imperious way, Craig had banished HIV from his psychological world—begone, unwanted interloper, don't trespass here! By dint of his self-granted authority, he steadfastly refused to let HIV interfere with his life and psyche. And so far, the virus had complied.

For men who adapt to HIV with a style of Impassivity, HIV only minimally disrupts their previous views of themselves and life. The most striking feature of their response is the lack of response. Despite being infected and acknowledging (intellectually) the fact of AIDS' massive impact, these men maintain their same basic sense of self-identity, their same fundamental beliefs about justice, fairness, spirituality and fate, the same attitudes about the purpose or meaning of life.

Impassivity is not the same as "passivity." Although Sam was rather quiet, neither he nor Craig took a passive approach to life, or to their self-care. Instead, Impassivity refers more to their seeming neutrality or imperturbability in the face of AIDS. They approached it dispassionately, without the sense of upheaval demonstrated by so many others.

These men do not struggle with the "Why?" of their situation. AIDS has not unleashed for them the existential nightmares that hound others; they do not need to search their souls to find sense in what is going on. Theirs is not the anguish of a worldview shattered. They do not ruminate on unanswerable questions that plague some of their peers: "How could this be? Why is this happening?"

In the interviews, the four men whom I came to see as having this type of reaction responded to a few particular questions in similar ways. When I asked how HIV had affected or changed them as people, they answered that it hadn't, or they offered changes that were relatively minor. Some shrugged off the question by assuming that any changes stemmed primarily from non-HIV-related maturation, and so probably would have happened anyway.

When I asked (all the men) if they could identify beneficial aspects of their situation, some waxed eloquently about their bittersweet growth; others envied benefits they saw in others but not in themselves. Among these men, the answers ranged from lukewarm Yes to equally lukewarm No. Sam and Craig's already quoted words capture this narrow response. For them, the question seemed not to make much sense.

Impassivity may appear the most perplexing of all the possible reactions to HIV. It seems shocking in its lack of shock, dramatic in its lack of drama. After all, adversity is expected to be traumatic. How can a person respond to something as monumental as AIDS by staying essentially unchanged?

In fact, this response may even go beyond perplexing some people. It may unsettle, threaten, disturb. This is particularly true for those who have experienced much greater emotional turbulence themselves; they assume others need to go through the same traumatic response. The pain of the trauma must be disguised or buried. People can't react to something this cataclysmic with benign indifference: The person must really be "in denial" or "blocking" a deeper reaction.

Perhaps. People certainly do block and deny. We spare ourselves from facing blunt truths, sometimes adaptively, sometimes harmfully. We may hide in a self-deluded world of deception, more readily apparent to others than ourselves.

But not always, and not all people. *Not everyone needs to go through great crisis to cope effectively with trauma.* It's not that such people are defensively fending off an underlying terror (as is the case with Camouflage). These are not men who are simply fooling themselves. It's more that their style of responding to major upheaval is to get (somewhat) upset, shrug their shoulders, sigh, and go on.

This may be a more widespread response to HIV than anyone suspects. For, in some ways, these are the men we know the least about. They are not as likely as others to show up in psychotherapists' offices, self-help groups, or activist organizations. They are less likely to picket, march, attend workshops, or participate in healing services. They are not trumpeted in media stories of courageous living. They do not write autobiographies telling us of their inspiring journeys. They do not proselytize their style of living with HIV. And they tend to be out as HIV-positive to fewer people, because their infection is a less central part of their personal identity.

This style may be harmful if it interferes with appropriate self-care or leads to engaging in dangerous behaviors. However, for some men Impassivity is the most adaptive response to dealing with the potentially massive trauma of HIV. As long as someone takes good care of himself and is not overly hindered by anxiety or depression, this style can be a viable strategy for maintaining the belief in a meaningful world.

HIV and Self-Identity

Perhaps Impassivity is most noticeable in the way HIV enters, or does not enter, a person's sense of who he is. Men with this style tend to downplay any identification with HIV. Jules's words at the chapter's beginning reflect this. He "consciously" chooses *not* to identify as a person who is HIV-positive. He does not want to include HIV as a central part of his identity.

This stands in sharp contrast to how many other HIV-positive gay men identify themselves. In fact, some men make a telling linguistic leap: They omit the word "positive" from the phrase HIV-positive. They refer to themselves as simply "HIV." They say things such as "I've been HIV since . . ." or "Others who are also HIV. . . ." It's not that men who adopt this language are necessarily equating themselves with, or reducing themselves to, the virus. Instead the phrasing indicates a tremendous degree of self-identification with HIV. For them, HIV is not something to keep compartmentalized: It has come to permeate, and to some degree define, their sense of self.

Some men go even further than this verbal leap. They mark themselves as infected by tattooing the phrase "HIV-positive" on their body.[2] Most often this is a political act—a bold way to confront others' fears and prejudice, and to undo the potential stigma of being positive by setting the terms in which it is defined. But just as telling as this political context, and the powerful role in life's meaning that such an act reveals, is how strongly these men mold their self-concept around HIV.

Men with a style of Impassivity, on the other hand, tend to minimize their infection so that it does not become a prominent factor in their identity. They do not call themselves "HIV," they do not tattoo their status on their arm. They do not rally around AIDS as a focal point in a newly evolving sense of self.

Nonreactivity to Change

If you ask some men when they learned they were HIV-positive, they'll tell you—exactly. Leon said, "April 30, 1989, 9:30 A.M." Eugene remembered not only the date, but what he was wearing. Stan and Nate heard it as a "death sentence." Willy reflected that it was "probably the worst day I ever lived through," and Leon "completely fell apart":

> I crumpled up in the chair and started to cry and came apart. I wasn't screaming, but I was crying. I remember covering my face with my hands; it felt like my whole world just fell apart. . . . I'm not a person who's given to drama, I don't like to be noticed at all, but when I left I couldn't do anything but walk up the street crying and babbling, it was awful. It's something I will never forget.

Such a pronounced response, and such precise recall, are not uncommon. The event marks the beginning of an extraordinary, unparalleled shift in life. As most people indicate, it "changes everything."

Yet some men describe a low-key reaction to learning they were infected, whether their positive test was expected or not. Sam's reaction was quite subdued. Such a calamitous event—and how mundane his response:

> Even though I expected it, I was disappointed. Some people go into a kind of a paralysis for a little while, but I didn't. I went to work that day.

Likewise, Craig treated it as humdrum news: "It was just confirmation. It wasn't really a big deal."

This nonreactivity to change also carries through to other aspects of living with HIV. For many men, coping with HIV takes a dramatic turn with the first signs of major illness in oneself, or a partner, or dear friend. This can be a juncture point as traumatic as initially receiving a positive test result — another crisis to face, but with higher stakes. But this, too, seems not to be the case for men with a style of Impassivity. They may remain unfazed by AIDS, even in the face of actual impact.

Recall Craig's nonchalant attitude about the potential reality of living with AIDS, even though his two previous lovers had both died. Similarly, Sam wondered if his low-key reaction to HIV stemmed from a sense that AIDS seemed quite far away:

Maybe at the point that I get sick I'll realize what the infection means. I'm at a point where it doesn't mean anything, because nothing has happened.

It may be true that serious illness would change Sam's reaction. But he must have been using a very narrow definition of the phrase "nothing has happened": Joseph, his lover, had AIDS. Joseph had already faced one bout of PCP (the infection then responsible for more AIDS deaths than any other), lost a good deal of weight, and had a T-cell count "around 40." Most people would probably say that quite a lot had happened, not "nothing." But Sam's style of minimizing AIDS was more powerful than the real intrusion that it already represented in his life.

As Sam pursued this topic during our interview, he further demonstrated his ability to distance himself from the reality of the situation. I asked him what it was like when Joseph first got sick:

It was depressing, but not for long. It increased his worry level, but I don't think he was hurt too badly psychologically . . . I don't think it affected me that much that I can remember. It was a very hectic time, and my work schedule was very tough, it was around Christmas time. He was supposed to have his kids here, and because of that, he couldn't. That was upsetting to him, but I don't think it bothered me—I didn't have time to get bothered all that much.

Again, Sam's non-reactive stance wins through. He greeted Joseph's illness with the same equanimity with which he met his own test result. I suspect he will respond similarly if and when he becomes ill—something akin to, "I'm surprised that I'm not responding more, but, no, it's not too bad."

Related to this, some men with a style of Impassivity tend not to recall details very well. Craig learned he was HIV-positive "maybe a year and a half, maybe two years ago. I don't remember exactly." His ex-lover died "two or three years ago, maybe three. I don't know." Jules remembered only minor details of his first year of being HIV-positive: "It seems like so long ago." The gist of Craig's dismissive response to HIV was succinctly captured in his mistrust of T-cell counts and prophylactic interventions: "If you feel fine, you're fine."

This lack of attention to detail is likely both cause and effect of this style of adaptation. If you do not register an event as traumatic, why should the details of it be memorable? At the same time, putting significant details of a potential trauma out of consciousness helps maintain the belief that all is the same and nothing has changed. It helps prevent something from becoming a trauma. If you don't remember it, there's no need to get alarmed.[3]

Hidden Pain

It would be false to portray Sam and Craig, or other men with this style, as completely devoid of underlying fear, pain, or anger. Although their primary response is to face HIV with equanimity, they are not completely without pain beneath the surface.

Sam remained basically unfazed by life's curves, including HIV. But he also used the defense mechanism "displacement" to voice hidden anxieties and express feelings he disowned in himself. At one point in the interview, he mentioned, in his even-tempered voice and unperturbed manner, that Joseph had recently started losing weight again. As he continued talking, he abruptly switched topics and criticized Joseph's buddy from the local AIDS service organization:

> Joseph seems to be losing weight again. [Pause] The sad thing to see is his AIDS buddy, the 52-year-old I was telling you about, he's

getting carried away. He mentioned he had anal sex the other day, unprotected. How can he do that? . . . I just wanted to punch him in the face for doing something like that, he should be smart enough to know better.

Perhaps it really is the buddy he'd like to hit. But more likely, it's Joseph, or himself, or God, and he displaces these feelings onto the buddy. Sam's response to HIV primarily *was* one of resignation—but small indications such as this suggest he was less resigned and dispassionate than he claimed to be.

Similarly, other men who display a style of Impassivity also tend to attribute some of their hidden emotional reactions to other people, using defense mechanisms such as displacement and projection.

I described Jules in "HIV as Isolation." Although his sadness and loss were palpable, Jules's larger style of adaptation to AIDS was Impassivity. HIV had neither triggered discernible growth in him, nor decimated his life or worldview. A shy, soft-spoken, sad man, he seemed to straddle a border between Impassivity and Rupture.

We can see these defense mechanisms at work in Jules's adaptation to HIV. Like Sam and Craig, he minimized the reality of HIV, but did not show the same nonchalance when directly faced with evidence of AIDS' impact. Such contact frightened him, and likely fueled his reluctance to interact with other men living with HIV or AIDS. He purposefully limited his involvement in the HIV world, and ended a dating relationship with a healthy-looking man he knew to be diagnosed.

This actual "escape" was yet possible for Jules: His life had thus far been free of AIDS losses, ill friends, declining T-cells, or any health impairments. His disregard of AIDS did not rely on the reality-bending sleight-of-hand used by Craig and Sam. But he shared with them the strong desire, or need, to confine HIV to a minimal role in his framework of meaning.

Yet tellingly, this quiet young man's most animated moment in our interview came at the very end. I had stopped asking all my "official" questions, and we were chatting amiably. In this post-interview conversation, he began talking about the few support group meetings he had attended. The intensity of his response surprised me, given the restrained tone he had used throughout:

It amazes me how many people I meet at these support groups are just—one guy in particular struck me as the kind of person who has always wanted a lot of attention from people, and when he found out he was positive, this was the ultimate way he was going to get it. He almost seemed excited and exhilarated by it; it was just amazing to me. He advocated basically telling everyone you encounter that you're HIV-positive. It made me angry, because he was presenting it that if you don't feel comfortable telling every single person you can, then you're not dealing with this very well, which I thought was weird. I was angry at him, and I'm not even sure what the source of that was.

Perhaps Jules' anger stemmed, in part, from having his response to HIV invalidated by this man — what gave him the right to tell me how to be HIV-positive? But, more significantly, I also heard in his words a secret longing to indulge in the kind of attitude he inveighed against (i.e., he was defending against using HIV as a strategy for attention). Jules, who explicitly told me "I don't define myself as an HIV-positive person," was projecting onto someone else a disliked and unwanted part of himself: his own unexpressed needs for sympathy, compassion, recognition, and attention.

Yet even with the acknowledgment of hidden pain, and the use of defense mechanisms to keep this pain at bay, it is not that men with this style base their adaptation to HIV on self-deception, as in Camouflage. Harris comes to mind here as another example of a man who seemed adequately attuned to his emotional responses to his situation, but for whom HIV had minimally affected his life's meaning.

In several ways, Harris differed from Jules, Craig, and Sam. To some extent being positive *had* become central to his worldview: "HIV affects the way I think about everything." Nor did he try to minimize contact with people with AIDS. In fact, he gave just the slightest hint of enjoying the emotional drama AIDS had created in others' lives. (This differed from Sam, who relished the momentary thrill of telling people about himself. Harris seemed more adept at using other people's adversity to enliven his own rather tepid sense of vitality.)

And yet, despite how it "affects everything," HIV had resulted in no significant overall change in Harris's psychological makeup. Harris had not by any means adapted poorly to HIV — but he gave several indications of having already adapted poorly to life. He coped well with HIV within this context, but AIDS had triggered no meaningful change.

Harris's life was one of disappointment and unfulfilled potential. Educated, bright, wealthy, and likeable, at 37, he had worked only as a desk clerk at an inexpensive motel. In his initial description at the outset of our interview, he said:

> I'm not very self-confident. I'm fairly bright, I'm kind, I'm a good friend. . . . I wouldn't want to sit here and let you think that I was well adjusted, because I don't feel like the world's best adjusted person . . . I just don't have a good sense of who I am.

Harris ached for a sense of purpose in life, something to rectify his sense that he was deficient. He cried as he watched television footage of American military heroism and camaraderie, because of the resolve demonstrated by the soldiers:[4]

> I thought it was really terrific to see all these people that were part of a group effort. . . . I don't think war is a glorious thing, but I was really touched by all these people, taken from their normal lives and thrown into this situation and achieving something.

Harris believed that living with HIV, facing AIDS, and coping with so much loss *should* be a catalyst for meaning. He wished there were something he could do, some organization he could join, to act on his altruistic yearnings:

> I would like to do something that makes a difference to someone before my time is over. But I don't know what that thing is. It would be terrific if we could come up with an organization for doing significant work for something in the little bit of time we have left. . . . I wish someone would come up with some organization with some wonderful mission, like taking us all to Romania to work with all those kids in orphanages, just to do something good.

It may come as quite a surprise to many other people that one needs to wait for an Eastern European relief effort for the opportunity "to do something good." Clearly, such opportunities exist just outside Harris's doorstep, as they do for everybody. But his desire "to do something good" was sharply at odds with the lack of purpose that long antedated his HIV infection. Harris struck me as a decent man who had not been able to make use of the inner resources he had, despite what he called the "stern mortal warning" of AIDS.

HIV had not rendered Harris psychologically impotent, nor had it jarred him out of the lifelong impotence that had long hampered his sense of initiative. Harris responded to AIDS with the same inability to mobilize his strengths that he had already repeatedly demonstrated, or failed to demonstrate. In the context of how Harris made sense of life and his place in the world, HIV was irrelevant.

I suspect that many people who have responded to HIV with Impassivity—in themselves, or regarding the epidemic as a whole—carry with them a nagging doubt: There's something the matter that I haven't reacted more strongly. Even though a low-key or minimal reaction may be what is most true to themselves, they face pressure from others, subtle or overt, to "really" face their feelings. And this pressure can be quite strong—from family, friends, peers, even therapists (unfortunately, in some cases, especially therapists). Individuals who deviate from social norms about how to face adversity can meet with reactions ranging from mild discomfort to frank disapproval.

Craig captures a piece of this distinction between his style of adaptation to HIV and others' expectations. He has no patience with the "outpouring of concern" voiced by family members, friends, and acquaintances:

> When people ask you how you are, they go, "How *are* you?" They'll ask you two or three times, and it's annoying. I say, "I'm fine, I'm not sick. How are you?" It's stupid, I don't like that.

By way of analogy, let's look again at grief. We have powerful cultural myths, usually unspoken, about how to mourn "correctly." These myths touch on many aspects of grieving—how long to mourn, what to feel, what not to feel, how to behave, how not to behave, when to show certain responses, with whom to share your feelings, and so on. Mourners face many implicit directives about how to conduct their grief.

But these myths are not always true. A growing mound of research suggests that many of our most basic, unquestioned assumptions about how people cope with loss may not match people's actual experiences.[5]

Many people (perhaps most) follow a similar path in grieving a major loss, at least in Western cultures. We respond with depression and pain for a discrete period (perhaps a couple of years), and then gradually return to our previous level of functioning. But a sizable minority don't follow this path. Some have a very prolonged reaction. Others have a very abbreviated one, regaining the full momentum of their life in quick measure. And to react differently from the cultural norm—by grieving too long, for example, or too little—needn't mean that a response is unhealthy. People vary greatly in how they respond to a significant life upheaval; the absence of turmoil may simply reflect another style of "normal" response.

This minimized response to loss is partly what I understand as Impassivity in the face of trauma. A person's overarching response to a significant adversity—the death of someone beloved, say, or HIV infection, or some other major personal upheaval—is to remain largely unchanged, unaffected. Despite the potential jolt to life's meaning, little actually changes in how a person sees his world. The adversity does not rankle or shatter. It does not inspire bittersweet growth. It quickly enters into the stream of life events with a surprisingly minor splash.

The fact that some men respond to HIV with this style raises the question of what it means to adapt well to trauma. Is this response a "good" thing? Are men who use this style coping well?

From one perspective, no, they are not. Minimization, denial, compartmentalization, displacement, projection, repression — a smorgasbord of defense mechanisms sustains this style. Some of these men (such as Sam and Craig) seem so indifferent to AIDS that it's hard to believe this can be healthy adaptation. Their nonchalance flies in the face of what "consensual reality" would have them recognize as indisputable facts in their lives.

Yet, when framed instead with the criteria of actual life functioning, the answer changes. Craig and Sam were both in ongoing romantic relationships (Craig's being the more satisfying). Each attended to his own health, despite keeping images of AIDS' illnesses far at bay. Neither reported any undue anxiety or depression. Craig saw a therapist intermittently, but felt no need to do so currently. Sam had actually derived self-esteem benefits from his newfound openness about his HIV status and homosexuality. Among the men I spoke with, these two engaged in the most reality-bending dismissal of their situation. Yet they also seemed to have adapted well to their lot.

Jules's adaptation, on the other hand, was less free of impairment. His a painful and isolated world. He did not like to be identified with HIV. He told very few people about his infection. A few months before we spoke, he began psychotherapy because of experiencing panic attacks and depression. His casting of HIV as unimportant to his self-identity seemed motivated by fear, and not an adaptive response to maintaining life's meaning in the face of trauma.

For some men, Impassivity reflects a stoic, nonemotional personality style that predates HIV. Others are depressed, or have had a long-standing belief in their own helplessness (HIV as confirmation of powerlessness). For still others, this style is more akin to a Zen-like acceptance, an equanimity that shapes their attitude toward life and the vagaries of fate.

So, on the surface, Impassivity is neither automatically "good" nor "bad," adaptive nor dysfunctional. It could be both, or either. In this regard, it is similar to Camouflage. Whereas Transformation seems clearly to indicate a healthy adaptation, and Rupture indicates difficulty coping, Camouflage and Impassivity are not so clear cut.

For some men, this is the most adaptive and true way to respond (I'd put Sam, Craig, and probably Harris in this camp). It is neither "better" nor "worse" than Transformation. It is an alternative style of resilience. For other men, however, such as Jules, the yearning to maintain an indifference toward HIV seems a brave, but tenuous, attempt at getting by.

Of course, judging the relative benefits of any pattern of adaptation can only happen in the ongoing, fluid context of a person's life. Meaning-making evolves, and none of these styles is static or frozen. For some men, Impassivity is a final destination, and a good one at that. Not for them the epiphanies of growth or the ravages of despair. But for other men, Impassivity is a way station on a road elsewhere.

And, as with the other men, I wonder what will happen if and when these men get sick. Based on how they described their present and past reactions, Sam and Craig, I assume, will remain psychologically unchanged. They already indicated ways in which this style transcended the details of their situation.

Harris might also stay the same, or perhaps actually finally discover within himself the courage to grow. He so loved other people's dramas of illness that the chance to play out his own infirmities might unleash strengths he has yet been unable to mobilize.

Jules (along with Francis, in Camouflage) is one of the men from the study I worry about. I fear he has the capacity to slip further into depression and isolation. To me, his sense of resignation conveyed not so much benign indifference as an anger and betrayal he felt unable to express. Impassivity fit into Jules's long-ingrained pattern of accepting life's travails, but without Sam's equanimity or Craig's grand, useful, arrogance.

As with the other styles, Impassivity is an abstraction — the distilled essence of a real response, but something often murkier in real life than theory. It can border on Transformation or Rupture. It can fluctuate with other styles. It can resonate as true in general, but with specifics other than those I describe—a self-assessment along the lines, "I've grown some, I'm hurting some. But what a surprise that things are still basically the same, as normal (or abnormal) as they've always been."

Impassivity is the reaction that most strongly contradicts our notions about how people face adversity. But perhaps the question worth exploring here is not, "Why are these men blocking their true feelings?" but instead, "How can we validate that this is one of the expectable ways people face a crisis?" For, in fact, research with a variety of traumatized populations — parents who have lost infants to Sudden Infant Death Syndrome, women who have been raped, people fighting cancer—indicates that this need not be an unusual response to facing potential trauma.[6]

No similar research has been conducted among people living with HIV. Several major studies of gay men, however, suggest that most HIV-positive individuals are coping at least well enough to get by.[7] Perhaps these studies include large numbers of men with this style of adaptation: those who have more or less accepted HIV into their established personal identity and view of life, without ruffling their feathers too much. Such men may constitute a silent majority of those living with HIV, an entire lot of men who lead lives not of quiet desperation, but of salutary acceptance.

Part Three

Restoring Meaning

8

Living with Uncertainty, Ambiguity, and Questions of Mortality

One of the greatest challenges of life with HIV is the uncertainty of it all. Distressing questions abound: Will I get sick? When? How? Am I prepared? With what ailment? What's the best way to take care of myself?

Tolerating the unknown can be extremely difficult, so it is not surprising that most people strive to reduce uncertainty in their lives—not only with major hurdles such as HIV but with minor day-to-day concerns as well. One way we do this is by establishing consistency in a multitude of small ways. We keep our housekeys in the same place (and feel annoyed or frustrated when we can't find them). We create a morning routine for starting the day. We water our houseplants weekly, or pay the bills monthly, or watch the same television show with regularity.

Of course these mundane matters are not at all on a par with acclimating to life with HIV. Yet such minor details, usually taken for granted, play a crucial role in the subtle unfolding and sustenance of life's meaning. We organize our lives to maximize a sense of regularity. We like things to be orderly, controllable, "knowable," to predict with accuracy what will befall us. We build for ourselves worlds that follow certain expectations. Contrary to Ralph Waldo Emerson's words, consistency is *not* the hobgoblin of small minds: It is a basic strategy for how we create meaning in life.[1]

People vary in how much consistency they like, or can muster. But, as a general rule, most of us prefer a life that is more-or-less orderly. We routinize and automatize what we can—to save time and foster an (often illusory) sense of personal control. We create lives that offer adventure perhaps, but more often stability and consistency as the mainstay.

AIDS, HIV—these are supremely ambiguous and uncontrollable events. Uncertainty becomes the primary backdrop against which life is played, not an occasional disruption. Too many of the basics, long assumed, can no longer be taken for granted. Too many questions go unanswered.

Some men adapt to HIV by embracing this ambiguity, tolerating or even relishing the uncertainty. This becomes part of a process of "letting go," of giving up the illusion of control. These men rebuild meaning by radically changing their assumptions about the certainty and predictability of life.

More commonly, however, people follow a more moderate course, and seek ways to reestablish a sense of control or "knowability" in their life and world. In small but significant ways, they search for strategies to lessen the ambiguity of being HIV-positive. The unconscious aim is to make their lot seem less random or chaotic—and thus less of a threat to a belief in the world as meaningful.

How do people tolerate or reduce the uncertainty of living with HIV? How does HIV affect thoughts about death, dying, and mortality? Both questions are central to maintaining meaning in life in the shadow of AIDS. Both influence the style—and effectiveness—of how people cope. And both exert their sway at a level that is most often beyond our awareness.

To a large extent, these two questions cut across the four styles of adaptation and the ten representations of HIV we have looked at. And so in addressing them we will take a short detour off the pathway that winds through the rest of the book.

Creating an Orderly and Knowable World

Scientific progress continually chips away at AIDS' enormous mysteries, but life with HIV remains hinged on unknowns.[2] Pressing questions still beg serious answers: Does HIV invariably lead to AIDS? What potential co-factors delay or worsen the extent of immune deficiency? What are the relative benefits of Western medicine or alternative healing practices? Life with the virus is inescapably rooted in these uncertainties.

But, perhaps surprisingly, many HIV-positive men have come up with answers to questions that are, more objectively, unanswerable. These answers are anchored, to varying degrees, in fact, logic, hope, and benevolent self-deception. And these self-determined answers are generated to strengthen a belief that the world can be seen as orderly and knowable.

People use several mental strategies to reduce the inherent ambiguities of living with HIV and resurrect the illusion of a knowable, predictable world. These strategies may not, in fact, make the world a more tractable or manageable place—but a person may come to perceive it as such.

Imagining Who Infected Me

For example, some HIV-positive individuals decide just who it is who infected them. This may be a plausible decision, borne from a careful assessment of one's sexual history. Jules comes to mind here: He was certain he was infected by one or both of the men who raped him. His lack of other experiences with anal sex, his ex-lover's testing HIV-negative, and the subsequent illness of one of these men support his assumption.

Frequently, the belief "I must have been infected by *him*" lacks a logical rationale, given the number of partners and amount of high-risk sex in someone's history. It is a fiction a person creates to lessen the intolerable ambiguity of not knowing.

For example, both Sam and Harris said that they did not spend much time speculating about who infected them. But later in the interviews, each revealed a specific fantasy of infection. They framed their words in a way that suggested they half-believed, half-disclaimed these scenarios:

Harris: It would be absolutely impossible to know [when I got the virus], but I have a feeling that I actually might know who I did get infected from. . . . There was a period soon after I moved to New York when I had night sweats, and if that's when I got infected, then I have a pretty good idea who I got infected with. Coincidentally, that person was the best sex of my entire life. . . . But, on the other hand, I had spent the summer before living in Provincetown, and had spent all my vacations before that in Key West.

Sam: I know a guy who spends a significant part of his time wondering who it was and blaming various people. I don't. [Later in interview] . . . sometimes, I wonder about somebody I screwed around with about that time . . . it reminds me of one incident. I was with a friend of mine in the bar and we picked up somebody else. He had just moved to Boston from Chicago. I sucked him off, and he was shocked that I went that far. . . . I was very excited, and I got carried away. About a year after that, I found out he was sick, so I figured that's why he was taken aback when I took him all the way, like I shouldn't have . . . [pause] But I don't dwell on it. I probably got it from more than one person anyway.

Nate relied on a detailed rationale for determining who infected him. Given the relatively small number of partners with whom he was anally receptive, his belief may be accurate — yet the intricacies of his logic suggest that his need to pinpoint this one person supersedes the details of his explanation:

I have in mind a person who I would like to think wasn't the person, but statistically, it could be: otherwise, it's my whole background, or this one person. . . . I met this guy from San Francisco. . . . We had unsafe sex, and I was on the recipient end of it, and I didn't realize he was playing unsafely, so I think I may have been infected by him. I met him once a year afterwards in San Francisco, and I've been unwilling to check if he's sick, or even if he's still alive. I suppose I could go to the phone book and see if he's still listed: that would be some indication. Let's see: that's six years ago, that could be 600 T-cells added to the 400 or 500 that I have now, it would put me back up into normal range, so it could work. But I don't dwell on it.

Given Nate, Sam, and Harris's sexual histories, their infection could have come from any one, or several, of various partners. Yet I suspect they derived an odd comfort from personifying the man who infected them. It made being positive less random, less unknowable. As Nate said, "It's my whole background, or this one person."

Also noteworthy are the specific sexual encounters that some men assume to be the source of their infection. Harris romanticized that the person who infected him was also "coincidentally . . . the best sex of my entire life." Sam remembered it as an encounter in which he was "very excited." And Nate cryptically hoped that the person he believed infected him, whom he described as "really hot," wasn't the one who actually did.

Each assumes some connection between his degree of lust or passion and the likelihood of infection. Here, too, we see shades of punishment—if I'm infected, it must have come from sex that was too good.

Yet in addition to punishment, just as striking is how each fantasy reduces the ambiguity or mystery of these men's situation. These beliefs, half subscribed to, half disclaimed, allow Nate, Sam, and Harris to think they weren't infected randomly in an undeterminable encounter. By speculating that a specific person was responsible for their infection, by tracing their HIV transmission to a particular sexual episode, they are attempting to make more knowable, tractable, and manageable one of the ambiguous aspects of living with HIV.

Along similar lines, a patient once told me that while attending a weekend retreat he was robbed of some jewelry, probably by one of the other retreat participants. He conceded he had no factual way of knowing who the thief was. But he secretly assigned blame, rightly or wrongly, to one particular person. As we spoke, it became clear that assigning blame to this particular individual eased his mind. It helped him cope with the ambiguity of the situation and maintain trust in the others — this was preferable to thinking that the thief could have been anyone at all.

Setting Milestones

With surprising directness, most (not all) of the men I spoke with thought it likely that they would develop AIDS. They anticipated the future much as they faced the present: with varying amounts of hope, realism, optimism, denial, and dread. Yet this variety of responses narrowed when I specifically asked what, if any, hypothetical time frame a person had before any serious impairment. One predominant pattern emerged: Almost all used easy, round numbers to estimate a period of remaining health.

Of course, it's commonplace for people to think in easy round numbers such as this, regardless of HIV. Job interviewers rarely ask, "Where would you like your career to be in seven years, three months?" Thinking in five- or ten-year segments helps organize complicated time projections. It is one of the seemingly irrelevant ways in which we reduce ambiguity and uncertainty in daily life.

With HIV, this process takes on an added feature. It allows people to contemplate an extremely distressing unknown quantity—the amount of time someone might face until illness or death—by reducing it to a more manageable piece of information. It is yet another of the ways, some grand, some small, that we attempt to balance feared reality and soothing illusion.

Despite the actuality of where someone was in terms of T-cells or any signs of debility, most men spoke in chunks of "five years" or "ten years." For some, this becomes a perennial, ever-replenishing five years. The news of their infection may be greeted like a "death sentence," but it then evolves into a perpetual five- or ten-year lease on life. So someone, two years into infection, may believe he's got ten more good years, and then still think, "ten more good years" three years down the road.

Other men devise a similar strategy. They don't think in terms of five years or ten years, but choose milestones in their lives as appropriate goals to aim for. Nate, who was 46 years old, and Lucas, at 40, wanted to turn 50. Nate called turning 50 "a little goal" and Lucas, whose fiftieth birthday would be in the year 2000, exclaimed, at once wishful and uncertain, it was "not impossible." Willy, at 34, and Harris, 37, were shooting for 40. Stan and Charles wanted to make it until the twenty-first century; as Stan put it, "I'm planning on being around for the millennium, because that's something I would like to see. A whole year and a half or two of parties." Vincent wanted to attend the college graduation of his niece, currently a high school senior.

Shooting for nearby milestones, thinking in five- or ten-year chunks— we do it in daily life. But, with HIV, framing time in measurable units serves the additional purpose of restoring order and regularity. And five to ten years seems a good strategy. Five years is long enough away to seem neither immediate nor imminent, yet close enough so as not to grossly distort the gravity of the situation. It is a way to balance HIV's being present yet distant, real yet not real.

Knowing People with AIDS

Contact with people with AIDS is a double-edged sword. On the one hand, it can be too upsetting or frightening, too real an intrusion into a needed sense of denial. Yet such contact may also be helpful. It demystifies the unknown, it reduces the uncertainty of what may happen. For some men, learning what might be in store for them, rather than facing an unknown future, is a source of relief. This was the case for Willy:

I remember when George was still alive, and the few times I saw Kent during his illness. When I was around them, it was frightening on the one hand, and strengthening on the other. I would see the illness, and that would frighten me, thinking this may happen to me. But on the other hand, I'd look at it and say, "Okay, this is what I may have to deal with someday, and where it was a big surprise and shock to them, I have the chance now to prepare myself for what may come." That's been important to me, because in the past two years, I have spent a great deal of time in preparation, getting my life in order so that when and if illness does come, my life won't be in total turmoil the way it was for them.

And for Harris:

When my boss Sean got sick, that was the first time I ever visited anyone with AIDS in the hospital. It was a very good experience for me to go there and see how he was treated, because I had heard all these nightmares about how AIDS patients were treated like pariahs, and that was not the case at all with Sean. In the hospital, he had the most remarkable set of nurses: they were terrific, they were funny, I was really touched by their kindness.

For Harris and Willy, having tangible evidence of what might lie ahead is helpful. What had previously been mysterious has been revealed, made visible. George, Kent, and Sean's experiences seemed disturbing, but they also provided a real image around which to plan and anticipate the future.

Not all men find this to be the case. Recall Jules's aversion to dating a man with AIDS, and his general reticence about being with other men who were positive. Vincent had never had any contact with a person with AIDS, and seemed in no great rush to do so. These men preferred keeping AIDS as far away as possible. Perhaps most men living with HIV have no choice in the matter—friends or lovers are (or were) sick. For them, contact with people with AIDS is unavoidable. These relationships contain a mix of support, sadness, dread, and inevitable comparison.

Yet despite the possible difficulties inherent in such contact, for some men knowing and seeing people with AIDS provides a helpful measure of internal structure. It allows them to begin to tolerate and prepare for might lie ahead.

Predicting the Likelihood of AIDS

Well into each interview, after we had established a trusting rapport, I eased into more sensitive topics. Among these, I was interested in hearing what the men thought the future held for them, and I asked directly what they thought the likelihood was of developing AIDS. Most said they were quite sure they would.

This did not apply to everyone. For some, thinking about moving from being HIV-positive to having an AIDS diagnosis was too distressing to contemplate. When this question came up for Leon, a sense of sudden anxiety clouded the openness and lucidity of the rest of the interview, even though he had calmly discussed topics that were (to my thinking) more distressing:

> That's a frightening question. I don't think about it. No, of course, I think about it all the time, but I don't get to the point of giving myself an answer like you want. What is the likelihood ... [Long pause] I'm having more trouble telling you that because it brings up all kinds of superstitions and anxieties. I can go into a spiel about statistics, which I think are bullshit—I know that it's a progressive disease—I can't give you an answer. I'm going backwards and forwards in my mind. ... The question makes me so anxious that I can't answer you.

A few other men, while not acknowledging their anxiety, also gave vague answers that seemed related to the frankness of the question. Craig said, "I haven't got a clue ... I have no idea, I haven't really thought about it," and Stan and Francis used the question as a springboard for their hopes that they might be personally exempt from AIDS.

Yet the clear majority of men thought it very likely that they would develop AIDS. Anthony, Sam, and Howard placed the likelihood at "100%." Nate put the probability at 90%, and Harris at 95%. Others simply expanded on themes such as "It's pretty likely," "It's very likely," and "I suppose it's inevitable." Most felt that they had some control, if not over the eventual outcome, at least over the onset of symptoms, either by taking

AZT and prophylactic drugs or through a health regimen of good diet, physical exercise, and regular sleep.

From one vantage point, for a person to expect that he will most likely develop AIDS seems reasonable—it jibes with scientific fact and the laws of probability. (It also probably reflects the media's misguided depiction of HIV as unfailingly leading to AIDS, and the equally destructive presentation of AIDS as inescapably lethal.)[3] Yet it also seems counterintuitive. Wouldn't it be more adaptive to believe that you will be among the statistical minority who stay healthy?

Expecting that AIDS is likely, while pessimistic, serves an important function. Like other mental strategies, it helps demystify the uncertainty of the situation. It turns the amorphous into the concrete. This may be preferable to the more optimistic, but far more ambiguous, stance of not knowing what the future holds.

Accepting the likelihood of developing AIDS does not mean abandoning hope. Perhaps by acknowledging the worst that might happen, we can paradoxically allow a deeper hope to flower.[4]

Taken at face value, these strategies of reducing ambiguity may seem odd, distorted, counterproductive. Imagining "I was infected by *him*" is often not only inaccurate, but suggests blame. Seeing one's life expectancy as a floating five to ten years seems simplistic. And anticipating "I will most likely develop AIDS" flies in the face of positive thinking.

Yet each of these distortions—illusions, yet again—serves a greater psychological need than the specific point at hand: inhabiting a universe that follows orderly rules. We prefer a world that is knowable rather than amorphous, one that is manageable, not random. By reducing the inherent ambiguities of life with HIV, these mental strategies help maintain beliefs in meaning.

Thoughts of Death and Dying

In the 1920s, a German literary and social critic, Walter Benjamin, wrote about the profound effect of modern medicine on how we deal with death:

> In the course of modern times dying has been pushed further and further out of the perceptual world of the living. There used to be

no house, hardly a room, in which someone had not once died. . . .
Today people live in rooms that have never been touched by death,
dry dwellers of eternity, and when their end approaches they are
stowed away in sanatoria or hospitals by their heirs.[5]

This is no longer true for gay men. With the advent of AIDS, death has
reversed its retreat "further and further out of the perceptual world of the
living." Death has catapulted forward, made itself dramatically present. It
looms as a grotesquely dominant feature in the landscape, or cityscape, of
our lives. Brunches and tea dances, once the stuff of Sunday afternoons,
have been eclipsed by "a relentless series of memorial services and funerals
— the new tribal rituals of life in the time of AIDS."[6] Bars and bathhouses, long the social fiber of urban gay life, compete for popularity with
agencies that tend the ill. In symbol and in reality, in our private homes and
our community structures, gay men's lives buck the singular most powerful
drift of Western twentieth-century civilization. We no longer inhabit rooms
untouched by death.

As might be expected, concerns about death and dying often become an
intrinsic part of living with HIV. "I think about death a lot," said Anthony.
"I'm sure I would not be thinking about it much at all if it weren't for
AIDS." Stan was far more hopeful than most that either luck or good genes
might grant him an exemption from AIDS, despite his declining T-cells. Yet
he too spoke of death's omnipresence in his thoughts:

> It's always there, because once you're told you have a death sentence
> hanging over you, you think about it at different times. It isn't a
> constant thing, you're not completely absorbed by it all the time.
> But when you're walking by yourself, you might think about it.

In his ministerial work, Lucas had witnessed death, and the process of
dying, among many friends and congregants. He had officiated at almost a
dozen AIDS funerals, all the while secretly bearing his own infection.
Regarding his own death, he said:

> I've taken it much more seriously, I've been with it more, thought a
> lot more about it. What dying is, what it's about, what it means,
> images of dying, how can dying become something that I can enter
> and be with. I've turned to my theology more and more to find out

how other people have wrestled with this, or viewed it or seen it. What has been most helpful has been the mystics, Judeo-Christian mystics. It remains a complete mystery to me. I don't know what death is, and I don't understand what happens after, but I believe there is a force of love, and there is a mystery that becomes revealed at some point. Death has become much safer than it ever used to be, it feels like it can be a safe place where one can turn over one's whole self, even the self that I've worked so hard to build can be held lovingly by this higher power. . . . Right now, I'm not hideously scared of it.

A few men—Lucas, Anthony, Kyle, and Victor—seemed determined to face thoughts of death squarely, fighting the deeply ingrained habit in all of us to shrink away from the topic. Kyle and Victor in particular saw this as a crucial aspect of living with HIV: preparing themselves for the spiritual journey they anticipated the process of dying to be.

Charles, although overcome with grief for the recent death of his friend Tony, worried less about his own death. He had attempted suicide as a young man. He felt he had been near death before, and gained a sense of calm from this experience:

When I was 23 or 24, I tried to commit suicide. I took about 20 Nebutols and drank a bottle of Kwell lotion, because somebody told me it was poisonous. Then I went into the bathroom, took a razor blade, and cut both my wrists. The only thing I remember about it was this beam of light, this Jesus-like figure with a beard, and this overwhelming sense of serenity for the first time in my life, an overall calmness. I remember him sort of shaking his head and saying, "Not yet." Not yet: when my time comes, it comes. That's what I hang on to, that feeling. It makes it more comfortable to think about dying. What lies beyond death, for me, is this warm, gentle feeling.

Victor spoke about death with a greater immediacy and intimacy than I have ever heard in anyone else, healthy or ill, young or old. Recall, from Chapter 5, his intense, reverie-like meditations on massage work with dying people. His words were infused with a powerful combination of horror and bravery.

I think Victor felt driven to confront his fears about death. He seemed to wrap himself in it, to push himself to the brink of imagining a truth he fearfully knew awaited him. He wanted to know as much as he could about it to prepare himself. His approach was part respect, part defeat, part submission, and part egoistic flamboyance—even with this, he was not going to be upstaged.

Yet while some men shared with me raw thoughts about their own death, most spoke about it only at a remove. Nobody admitted to actually being scared of death—Leon's anxiety to my asking about the likelihood of developing AIDS seemed certainly to touch on this, but he did not address it directly. Instead, most of the men spoke about dying in a level voice, betraying neither fear nor loss, as if it were an event that would happen to somebody else. A common refrain was, "I don't really have a fear of death—but I do fear the process of dying." In other words, while the men spoke with detachment about death, fears about illness were prevalent.

AIDS has unlocked a Pandora's box of medical anomalies and diseases. A range of specific horrors may lie in store—physical disfigurement, blindness, mental dysfunction. Like an evil grab bag from a party in Hell, people have particular fears of which unwanted gift they may be forced to bring home. Many people report that a fear of these infirmities troubles them more than the fear of death itself.

Other issues related to death and dying are also a source of worry: Will people be there to help take care of me? Is my partner strong enough to handle this? Will I become destitute? Can I handle becoming incapacitated, losing my independence, becoming a burden? How will my death affect those I love, and who love me?

Sam worried what would happen if he and his lover became debilitatingly ill at the same time — and what were the "relative advantages" of dying first or second? Charles feared several scenarios: watching his lover (who was also HIV-positive) die, becoming a "vegetable," and, most distressing for him, losing his "dignity" and "values" as he struggled through illness. Anthony, who had recently started dating another HIV-positive man, admitted it was "kind of hard to fight the sense of 'Why am I bothering at this point to have a relationship, since I'm only going to get sick and die?'"

In addition to these acknowledged fears, concerns about the potential of illness and death surfaced in the interviews in two additional ways. First, many of the men cried or became teary at some point in the interview—

sometimes when talking about grief, but, more tellingly, at less weighty moments. Someone may have spoken calmly about a fear of facing blindness or dementia, but moments later started crying when discussing giving up sweets to improve his diet.

Of course, this phenomenon occurs outside the interviews as well. I asked many of the men when, and if, they cried. By far the most common answer was that they did cry, but infrequently, in private—and usually in response to such cues as pop songs, news stories about strangers, melodramatic movies, or mawkish, overblown television commercials.

Here again the defense mechanism "displacement" is at work. These brief releases of emotion allow people to channel their fears away from truly anxiety-provoking material and vent them on safe topics, where they can exert more control. The tears we shed watching a sappy commercial are not about the commercial itself; they adaptively funnel emotion into a more innocuous outlet. They allow us to express sorrow and grief for pain too difficult to address head-on.

Second, the terrible reality of AIDS can sometimes abruptly intrude into daily life with an unexpected, forceful presence. This happened in the interviews several times. Disrupting the surface calm of a more placid discussion, a sudden burst of graphic imagery would rip into the conversation. Leon's explicit discussion of his first AIDS patient, Charles's detailed description of his friend Tony's illness, Howard's unexpected tears when he told me his five all-time favorite sexual partners "were all dead"—all were intrusions of this sort. Unleashed with little or no warning, these vivid images quickly, ferociously, altered the tone of the interview from one of relative detachment to one in which the horrors of AIDS were momentarily fully present.

This also occurred with Franklin, the formerly homeless man who had found in HIV a great catalyst for growth. Franklin took our interview very seriously: He used it to mark his accomplishments but also to berate himself over his continued indulgence in anonymous, unsafe sex. Yet throughout he maintained a wry, wistful sense of humor, an awareness of the perversity of fate in how HIV had beneficially turned his life around.

For years, Franklin had lived on the streets—hustling, alcohol, drugs, "the whole nine yards." A "spiritual awakening" after testing positive two years earlier helped him quit drinking. Getting sober then led him to stop hustling and stay off the streets. He began to gain a long-neglected sense of self-respect. When we spoke, he was volunteering at an AIDS organization, speaking to poor, inner-city youths about HIV. He felt a sense of belonging and community that was new to him. He had plans to move out of the halfway house where he lived into his own apartment.

Humorous and brimming with pride over his accomplishments, Franklin kept the actual threat of AIDS far from his awareness—both in the interview and, I suspect, through much of his daily activity. But in the following story his voice grew somber. As he told me about his AA sponsor, a man who had been a tremendous role model for him, his protective distance from HIV evaporated:

> I chose him to be my sponsor because we have a lot in common—
> he's wild, I'm wild, he's a slut, I'm a slut. Well, he has full-blown
> AIDS. I chose him because I liked his spirit, his spunk, his desire to
> go on, to live in spite of. . . . He has fought as long and as hard as he
> could, and now he can't fight anymore. It's like the virus is winning
> now. [Here his manner begins to change.] He has dementia, and he
> has it bad. He's out there in left field, and I'm sure he's not coming
> back. To talk to him is like, man—it wears me out, it really wears
> me out. I was in his apartment when the cops came to get him: they
> was locking him up because of things he'd done. He was sleeping
> out in the hallway instead of his apartment, he had barricaded the
> door the night before and he had gone off in there, he was threat-
> ening tenants. He was up on the 14th floor, and he threw dirt and
> plants out the window. It was icing on the cake when I went to see
> him: he had climbed up the window and was threatening to jump.
> To see him like that, it was like he did a 360-degree turn. It just
> wore me out.

Franklin had spent most of the interview talking about what he saw as the "unreality" of AIDS. Only in the above passage did its reality, evoked in graphic details, come out. The image stood in sharp relief to all else he had said, and seemed suddenly to enshroud our meeting in the full brunt of his sorrow. In that moment, describing his sponsor may have been as sobering for Franklin as giving up alcohol.

Ironically, some men experience this kind of intrusion on a daily basis, in the process of caring for themselves. Taking AZT or another treatment may momentarily bring the sharp awareness of AIDS into the daylight. Leon spoke about this, as did several others:

To take lots of pills each day, it's such a drag. I can't help seeing the color of the pill and the whole mindset comes back. Maybe some people can do it and go on, but for me it brings it all back, even for a few seconds. And then I go on.

Lucas offered a moving example of how he was jarred into realizing the distance he usually kept between his everyday life and fears of his own death. He was meeting with a dying friend to prepare a eulogy for the friend's funeral. The friend did not know that Lucas was also HIV-positive:

Last summer, I went to see him about the service. He was getting weaker and weaker. There were a number of things I presented: Would you like this to be said, or that. There's one poem, a haiku . . . "I had always known that one day I would take this road. But yesterday, I did not know it would be today." That's what HIV has been for me: I've never denied death, the reality that my life is limited, but I didn't know it would be so soon that I'd have to come to terms with all this stuff. . . . Lee said "No, that's not accurate. I knew that this has been coming. AIDS is a terminal illness." A terminal illness. That was very hard for me, I had to close myself down. . . . It was with me for months. That was very painful, devastating in a certain way.

But as if to undo yet again the devastation of that thought, to re-invoke the necessary distance that helped him so much, he paused and went on, "I still don't think AIDS is a terminal illness, I don't, I don't."

The men also expressed thoughts about death and dying in their spiritual beliefs. As already discussed, many made reference to an afterlife, or a sense of ongoing community, or some belief that revealed a fantasy of symbolic immortality. Specific or vague, a source of solace or puzzlement, the idea that something of our life continues beyond death can be a helpful, perhaps necessary, support. Nate worried out loud that he would die alone and be forgotten. He added, quietly, "I sometimes think I should design my own quilt patch."

Related to these concerns about immortality, several of the men told me of their disappointment that they had no children, particularly sons. This was not something I asked about, yet it surfaced in several interviews.

Stan and Franklin, after learning they were HIV-positive, both said they needed to grieve the lost possibility of having a family. For Eugene, "the only problem I've ever had with being gay is not being able to be a father." He admitted, as if mildly embarrassed, that he was upset because he was "the only son of an only son, and so the name will go away with me." Not that any of these men had earlier acted on these desires of fatherhood: Neither Stan, 48, nor Franklin, 31, had ever had sex with a woman or pursued alternative paths to fatherhood. Other men — Anthony, Howard, Stan, Kyle, Eugene, and Vincent — all spoke of pleasurable relationships with younger men. These relationships were sexual, avuncular, or mentoring. They symbolically captured aspects of a father-son relationship.

In other words, for some men facing mortality gives birth to a fantasy, perhaps previously hidden or unconscious, of fathering a child. For men who have at times consciously explored fatherhood, HIV can nudge this belief into prominence, by dint of its no longer being an option.

On a conscious level, then, most of the men I spoke with contemplated dying and death from a necessary distance, through a veil of cognitive detachment. Fears of death were voiced in less direct ways—by displaced demonstrations of emotion, by identification with sick individuals, by pragmatic concerns about illness, and by the periodic sudden intrusion of graphic images of AIDS into an otherwise tranquil state of mind. Although some men strive to contemplate death with a minimum of facade, or to transform death's imminence into an impassioned challenge to live more fully, an awareness of death is more frequently acknowledged and granted respectful attention, but quite purposely underplayed.

In words that echo those of Walter Benjamin, Victor lamented how death is shunted aside in modern life:

> The world that we live in here doesn't have, hasn't yet made room for, dying. It's really odd, because it's something that everyone does. It hasn't even made room for people being ill. But if people start tending and caring for those who are obviously sick, maybe we can all start to grow, in a larger context. . . . We're all in recovery from something, dealing with some type of issue or problem. We all need healing.

Lucas interspersed our talk with poetry. He came to our interview armed with several poems that he had found helpful in coming to terms with HIV. Many were of a spiritual nature, in keeping with the essence of how he found meaning in life. But some also reflected doubt, uncertainty, and fear.

He ended our meeting by reading to me a poem by Czeslaw Milosz, "The Thistle, The Nettle":

> The thistle, the nettle, the burdock, the belladonna
> Have a future. Theirs are wastelands
> And rusty railroad tracks, the sky, silence.
>
> Who shall I be for men many generations later?
> When, after the noise of languages, the award goes to silence?
>
> I was to be redeemed by the gift of arranging words
> But must be prepared for an earth without grammar,
>
> For the thistle, the nettle, the burdock, the belladonna,
> And a small wind above them, a sleepy cloud, silence.

9

Coping, Changing, Growing

To cope effectively with HIV is to embrace opposites. The goal is to balance denial with self-examination, illusion with actuality, rebellion with acquiescence, risk-taking with safety. Accepting fate needs to be tempered by refusing to accept. Seizing control must be offset by relinquishing it.

Problems with coping can take many forms. People give up, or give in, or fight too fiercely, or escape too easily. Although they show different faces, these coping failures all share the same root: The interdependence of opposites has been lost.

Yet how difficult this balance can be to maintain, and how easy to career off course in a single direction. Some lose their way with too great an investment in illusion, others with too unflagging a confrontation with reality. Some fight to regain a control that can never be attained. Others prematurely dismiss all attempts at control as futile.

At best, these coping difficulties impede growth. At worst they cause danger or serious harm. Men who opt for too much illusion and too little reality risk shoddy self-care and inadequate preparation for the future; those who find no escape from reality may teeter into rage or suicidal despair. Searching for elusive control invites continual frustration and the possibility of addiction. Yet abandoning all attempts at control results in an unnecessary loss of inner vitality.

The great challenge of living amid HIV and AIDS is to discover a personal middle ground where these contradictions and opposites can co-exist. But how are we to get there?

I recall a fable from my childhood. The sun and the wind have a long-standing rivalry. Each believes he is more powerful than the other. One day they put their rivalry to the test. The competition: A traveler, ambling through the countryside, wears a cloak and hat as his outer garments. Who, the sun or the wind, will be more skillful at removing them?

The wind, gleeful, goes first. He feels certain of victory. The cloak hangs loosely around the man's shoulders. The hat is untied. Both can blow off easily. And so the wind begins to gust.

But as the gusts strengthen, the traveler wraps the cloak more tightly around him. He secures the hat to his head. The wind responds by trying harder: howling, bellowing, blowing ever more fiercely. Yet the harder the wind blows, the more tightly the traveler clutches the cloak to him, the more firmly he secures his hat.

The sun then takes his turn. With the wind spent, the sun steadily warms the fields in which the traveler walks. The day becomes calmer, the weather more clement. The traveler soon takes off his hat, and then loosens and removes his cloak. In short time, the sun accomplishes what the wind was unable to do, despite great effort.

This tale has become central to my understanding of how people change and cope—and how we frequently falter in our efforts to do so. In times of stress, we tend to act like the wind. We respond to an impending threat with a fierce attack—we cannot stand by and do nothing.

Sometimes this frontal attack works, in appropriate measure. But often it only worsens the situation. The cloak of our defenses, or our fear, anger, or maladaptive behavior, gets wrapped tighter. The harder we try to fight something, the more we may end up in its grip.

I believe this guiding principle of change runs counter to how most people go about it: To cope with an unwanted situation, strive first not to change it, but to accept it.

————————)-

What *is* coping? We use the word all the time—but what is it, what does really it mean, how does it work?

Perhaps the most detailed psychological explorations of coping come from psychologists Richard Lazarus, Susan Folkman, and their colleagues.[1] Drs. Lazarus and Folkman define coping as a person's ongoing efforts to "manage specific external and/or internal demands that are appraised as taxing or exceeding the resources of the person."[2] These efforts may include behaviors (active steps that you take), thoughts (mental strategies to help face or redefine stress), or a combination of the two. Coping is effortful, rather than passive or automatic. It is a process, not a specific trait or activity. And it is independent of outcome — that is, it may be helpful or harmful, successful or unsuccessful, effective or ineffective. Coping need not imply mastery over a situation, but simply an attempt to manage it.

Coping starts with seeing a situation as stressful. If a situation is not viewed as a threat, there is no need to cope with it. If two people face the same challenge but one sees it as a threat and another does not, their responses will differ.

Of course, people interpret HIV in a variety of ways, as reflected in the representations and styles of adaptation already described. Some men see HIV as a challenge to live more fully: their coping is shaped by the assumption that they can (or must) rise to a challenge. Others regard HIV as an inevitable mortal threat: Why bother to cope effectively if the outcome is certain? Still others appraise HIV as a nonstressful event, either by quickly resigning themselves to it or mentally postponing the need to register it as a threat until some later time.

In addition, Lazarus and Folkman also identify two primary types of coping: problem-focused coping and emotion-focused coping.

The aim of *problem-focused coping* is to change a stressful situation. Someone assumes that a situation can be altered, and that he or she is not helpless in changing it. With problem-focused coping the central question is, "What can I do, what steps can I take, to change the thing(s) that cause my stress?" Taking care of diet and sleep, seeking suitable health-care providers, or leaving a distressing relationship or job are all examples of problem-focused coping.

The aim of *emotion-focused coping*, on the other hand, is to lessen the psychological turmoil of unavoidable stressful circumstances. It focuses not on changing an anxiety-provoking situation, but acclimating to it. With emotion-focused coping, the main question is, "How can I change *myself* to deal with an unwanted situation?" Kyle captures the essence of emotion-focused coping in his stance toward HIV:

> I know that I'm not getting away from this. It's real, it's here, inside, and how I choose to deal with it is key. . . . I've never had a very strong sense that I could get rid of this, heal myself that way, but I *do* have a strong sense that I can heal myself spiritually and emotionally.

In daily life, with a range of stressful situations, we use a combination of problem- and emotion-focused coping strategies. We try to find ways to alter or curtail unnecessary stressors (problem-focused coping), but also accommodate ourselves to the reality of needing to live with some stress (emotion-focused coping). Ideally, in situations that can be changed, problem-focused coping should predominate. In situations that can't, emotion-focused coping results in a better overall adaptation. So although most coping responses involve a mix of the two, emotion-focused coping moves more to center stage in situations less amenable to change.

Do these principles of problem-focused and emotion-focused coping apply to HIV and AIDS? To a large extent yes, but not completely.

First, the yes. In good measure, these ideas continue to offer a valuable framework for understanding how to cope with AIDS. In all but the most calamitous circumstances, we can usually still find ways to make decisions and exert some control—that is, to use problem-focused coping. Even as emotion-focused coping needs to become more prominent the more extreme and unalterable the situation, problem-focused coping need never disappear.

Yet in other ways, these principles of problem- and emotion-focused coping may not apply. Extreme life situations are fundamentally different from the day-to-day problems of living, because massive adversity may completely destroy the framework we need to find meaning in life.

For example, studies of prisoners in Nazi concentration camps show evidence of both problem- and emotion-focused coping. Alas, they also show the failures and limitations of coping, the uselessness of tried-and-true strategies when an adversity we face is too great.[3] Coping can only occur in the context of a salvageable framework of meaning. For some concentration camp victims and survivors, and for some in the AIDS crisis, that framework has been shattered to the extent that typical coping strategies seem irrelevant and beside the point.

With HIV, coping begins, first and foremost, by simply carrying on with the daily tasks of living. A person cannot thrive without first surviving. Maintaining an ability to work, relating to others, just getting by—all are significant accomplishments. Rising above despair is a worthy achievement. Making the internal psychological leap from "dying of AIDS" to "living with AIDS" is no mere wordplay: Surviving in the face of potentially overwhelming trauma takes courage, faith, persistence, and tenacity. This is a great feat.

Of course, details of coping are not the same for everyone. No one-size-fits-all regimen will work. But by forging a middle-ground balance between opposites, by finding a mix of emotion-focused and problem-focused coping, a person can cope effectively with HIV and continue to find life meaningful.

No quick steps or magic formulas automatically lead to this resurrection of meaning. One of the most crucial (and sometimes frustrating) lessons of psychotherapy is that change cannot be forced or dictated—it must emerge from within. What a comfort it would be if we could find a handy guide to predict and organize our life's journey. But what a misrepresentation it would be to offer one.

Too many "how-to" books of psychological well-being — whether about living with HIV, repairing damaged self-esteem, recovering from abuse, or changing compulsive or self-defeating behaviors—offer the false promise that pain can be neatly healed. It can't be. A misguided search for easy answers may even go beyond not helping, and cause harm. Putting too much faith in quick-fix solutions can lead to greater disappointment and hopelessness.[4]

Still, certain coping strategies can help create the right kind of climate to foster change. Instead of regarding these as "how-to" steps of coping, we may more accurately regard them as laying a foundation conducive to growth.

By analogy, imagine wanting to attract a certain species of rare bird to your backyard garden. Assuming the general geographical conditions are right (i.e., the bird can be found in your region), you must then take appropriate steps: buying a specific kind of feeder, determining the appropriate location for it, using the right kind of food, finding ways to discourage predators, and so on. Following all these steps increases the likelihood that the desired bird will visit the garden. You still have no guarantee that the bird will come—yet not taking these steps all but assures that it won't.

The same is true in a journey of meaning. Taking certain steps may help you move along in the process. These steps offer no guarantee that growth will take place. Yet not taking them perpetuates the likelihood that growth will not occur.

Creating this foundation involves starting to do certain things and refraining from doing others. New behaviors or styles of emotional response may need to be learned. Obstacles that impede the path—maladaptive patterns, long-ingrained habits—may need to be cleared away. Some factors that may help create such an environment are increasing and deepening your social network; reexamining the notion of "control" in your life; attending to pragmatic health and life issues; developing distractions; curtailing addictive behaviors; and learning how to balance acceptance with fighting.

Let's look at these in more detail.

Increasing and Deepening Your Social Network

In Transformation, we saw the importance of community belonging among men who had adapted well to HIV. By reaching out to others, we create an environment conducive to growth. Feeling more connected to other people can be a central pathway to reestablishing meaning in life.

Strengthening your social network provides fertile soil for growth in several ways. Communicating with others improves the odds that you can be understood or heard, less isolated in pain. Behaving altruistically—doing volunteer work, participating in community organizations—can enhance self-esteem and provide a sense of purpose or accomplishment. And feeling part of a community is a means to redefine our existence—I am not just an individual, but part of something larger, a greater entity.

The "others" you connect with may be friends, family, lovers, a psychotherapist, a church group, a volunteer organization, an HIV-positive support group, a bowling team, a choir. It may be one individual or 20. It may be people you have known for years or new folks met through facing HIV.

Obstacles that may hinder your ability to reach out to others need to be recognized, addressed, and ideally worked through. For example, a sense of shame or stigma, fear of losing control over privacy (about HIV or being gay), worry that explaining your HIV status will be too emotionally draining—all these potential impediments to connecting with others warrant close examination. Do they hurt more than they help? What is their benefit, what are their costs?

One particular stumbling block to connecting with others is the belief that "nobody can understand." Perhaps this belief, more than any other, leads to a sense of isolation and disconnection. For some people, it is the greatest hindrance to feeling a bond with others.

Perhaps it's true. Perhaps nobody really can understand someone else's experience—with HIV, with any great pain, even with any day-to-day matter. Perhaps "I know what you're going through, I know what you're feeling" is always false. Maybe the poet John Donne was wrong when he wrote "No man is an island"—maybe we are all islands.[5]

But maybe we are not. Others may understand, they may not—but what is true is that *believing* people won't understand often becomes a self-fulfilling prophecy. If you assume that your experience cannot be understood by others, you are apt to perpetuate a sense of isolation.

In the past several years, researchers have learned a great deal about how we register incoming information from the world around us. A consistent finding emerges: As a general rule, people seek to confirm what they already believe, and dismiss or ignore information to the contrary.[6] In other words, it is much easier to strengthen our pre-existing ideas than to change them, because we don't look at all the evidence equally. In this way, believing "nobody can understand" can actually stop you from feeling understood. To the extent possible, challenge this belief, explore why you hold it, and find ways to muster the faith to counter it.

Reexamining the Role of "Control" in Your Life

We return yet again to personal control, one of the linchpins on which many of us hinge our framework for life's meaning. HIV need not lead to abandoning this belief completely—doing so may not even be possible. But effective coping involves examining and redefining it in ways that suit a changed reality.

This self-examination involves looking at the illusory and exaggerated sense of control most of us carry—and then finding ways to say goodbye to it. This does not mean bidding farewell to all aspects of taking control, but rather dismissing its monolithic, unquestioned prominence in how we create meaning. Absolute control is an unattainable goal. Pursuing it is responding like the wind in the fable.

A more adaptive strategy is to assess, more realistically, the specifics of what we can and cannot control. The notion of absolute control may be illusory, but much still can be under the sphere of your influence.

In the language of problem-focused versus emotion-focused coping, reexamining the role of control involves determining what can be changed and what can't. What are the things you can still exert control over (problem-focused coping)? What instead requires a change in internal attitude (emotion-focused coping)?

You cannot control having contracted HIV. You cannot control having suffered losses, or needing to prepare for more. You cannot control how other people will behave, who your parents or siblings are, or whether life is fair. You cannot control why your boyfriend is not perfect or why God did this to you. You cannot control anything that has happened in the past. Attempting to control these things is only to invite failure.

But you can control important life decisions, current and future. Whether to disclose your HIV status, when, and to whom. What health care choices seem most suitable—traditional or alternative methods, what kinds of prophylaxis, ideally the selection of a physician. You can control key decisions within the doctor-patient relationship. You can control your emotional and interpersonal patterns to a greater extent than often seems likely. You can control what goals to pursue, how to allocate your time, whether or not to pray. The options vary and may be limited by environmental, health, or economic circumstances. But the sphere of what you can control may be far wider than you think.

Bear in mind that believing in personal control is not necessarily desirable in and of itself. No abstract universal truth dictates "Seize control." Instead, maintaining a sense of personal control is valuable to the extent that it helps resurrect meaning. Control is one of the main ways we create meaning in Western culture; finding balanced ways to perpetuate this belief may provide threads of continuity in life.

Some individuals favor a different resolution. They attempt to catapult the notion of personal control from their life, seeing it as a misguided concept that has failed them. If this is driven from a sense of despair or defeat, it represents a failure of coping and an acknowledgment of meaninglessness. But if it follows from a conscious questioning of the value of control, and happens in the context of maintaining personal and interpersonal safety, it need not be a detrimental coping strategy.

Again, the primary underlying need is to maintain a framework for life's meaning. Most people will undertake this by seeking strands of continuity in their days, searching for beliefs they can maintain in the face of hardship. But some will start afresh with dramatically altered assumptions about life.

Addressing Pragmatic, Nitty-Gritty Issues

You also need to attend to pragmatic concerns regarding health, finances, and potential illness. Health-care proxies, living wills, a final will and testament, health and life insurance, support care networks, financial planning—all these issues become crucial.

Addressing some or all of these may be difficult for some people. Acting on such starkly real matters may violate a taboo of magical thinking —"How can I buy a cemetery plot? Isn't that admitting I'm going to die, giving up hope?"

No. "Hope" can be distinguished from a magical fantasy of special exemption. Perhaps true hope can only co-exist with pragmatism. Acknowledging the real possibility of illness may be frightening, but it can also allow you to discover new depths of inner strength. An unwavering and unrealistic belief in magical exemption from AIDS may be soothing for a time, but it doesn't allow you to know your real mettle.

True personal growth—with HIV or any other serious illness or trauma—is grounded in accepting the reality of the situation. And that reality typically involves facing a slew of unpleasant, but necessary, details.

Among these details, several categories of planning are most important: finances (present and future); health care; interpersonal support or assistance; arrangements related to illness or incapacitation; and desires or wishes related to burial, cremation, funerals, or memorial services. These don't all have to be addressed at once, or immediately. And seeking guidance or help from a local AIDS organization, and suitable professionals, can help you think about the specifics. But attending to these difficult pragmatic issues is as important as taking care of yourself emotionally and physically.

Getting Addictive Behaviors Under Control

Alcohol, drugs, sex, food—all these can provide a facade of coping. They offer temporary relief from intolerable feelings of loneliness, anger, or dread. They grant respite from frightening ruminations about mortality and illness.

In small doses, such diversion may be of great benefit. But if relied on too heavily, addictive and compulsive behaviors represent a failure of coping. They are not a viable strategy for handling stress. Perhaps soothing at the moment, compulsive behaviors can grossly impede real personal growth or the search for meaning.

As coping strategies, overreliance on alcohol, drugs, food, or compulsive sex leads to failure in two regards.[7] First, the behavior can become a serious problem in itself. A vicious cycle develops: If you drink, eat, or cruise to cope with stress, and the behavior itself becomes a source of stress, habit leads you to engage in more (not less) of the unwanted behavior. Addictions easily spiral out of control because of this, becoming both symptom and problem, gnawing away at self-esteem.

Second, compulsive behaviors arrest the formation of more adaptive responses. They not only become problems themselves, but they preclude the development of healthy self-esteem, competency, or resilience. They do not accrue any benefit. They are impediments that need to be cleared away so that more useful coping strategies can gain a foothold.

Altering addictive or compulsive behaviors may be a great struggle — typically, these are entrenched patterns not easily silenced. Yet learning to master or overcome an addiction can also be one of life's most transformative experiences. For several of the men I've described—Anthony, Franklin, Francis—getting alcoholism under control was a crucial turning point. Had they not gained mastery over their addiction, they would not have been able to approach the deeper life meaning each had come to savor.

In creating an environment conducive to personal growth, compulsive behaviors may be the greatest obstacles that need clearing. In our metaphorical garden, they are overgrown weeds, choking out all other flowers trying to grow. Popping up occasionally here and there, the weeds are manageable. Unattended, they ruin the possibility that one can find sense, order, or beauty in the land.

Developing Distractions

In the 1980s, David Feinberg wrote two vivid novels about life amid AIDS, *Eighty-Sixed* and *Spontaneous Combustion*. In *Queer and Loathing*, a posthumously published nonfiction collection, he wrote of his own experiences. He described HIV in his life, and the inescapable awareness of AIDS in his thinking:

> No matter what I do or think, AIDS remains the subtext, the subliminal humming of that perpetual-motion machine with six

rechargeable Energizer batteries hidden in the base. AIDS is always in the background, constant as the beating of my heart. If the virus itself hasn't yet passed the blood-brain barrier, the idea of the virus has already poisoned my mind.[8]

For some people living with HIV, the idea of developing distraction from AIDS is absurd. It's always there, at times glaringly bright, at times a "subliminal humming." Asking them to find distractions is no more realistic than asking them to change their fingerprints.

Yet discovering nondestructive ways to gain respite from AIDS-related concerns can be a great asset in coping with HIV. Learning how to do so can let you meet the challenges before you with more strength and courage.

Distraction may mean engrossing yourself in work. It may be finding suitable outlets of play. It might mean investing your time in a particular project or hobby, planning and taking a trip to a far-off locale, or getting involved in the details of planning an elaborate party. It can be writing a book, taking music lessons, studying t'ai chi, collecting stamps, building model airplanes.

Learning ways of distracting ourselves from pain, physical or emotional, gets bad press. Perhaps its value is maligned because it threatens cultural notions of what it means to be "strong." People should face their pain —to run away from it is "weak." But escape is a useful, undervalued coping mechanism. And the two needn't be contradictory. Admitting the reality of our pain doesn't mean that respite from it isn't possible or desirable.

Moving Toward Acceptance

Finally, creating an environment in which growth may flourish involves striking a new balance between fighting and acceptance.

This returns us to the fable of the sun and wind. In coping with HIV, a common but inadequate strategy is to fight against the changed and changing realities of life. This is to react like the wind. Paradoxically, the sun may make more sense.

In Western cultures, we learn from early on that giving in to a threat, not fighting it, is a sign of weakness or capitulation. Not to fight must equal giving up. Not to respond with force is seen as giving in.

But fighting certain things may only leave you more entrenched in them. You may of course yearn to rid yourself of the pain of HIV, or feelings of rage, despair, or fear; all these interfere with an ability to cherish life. But you cannot will them away. Accepting something does not mean you do not want it to change. It simply acknowledges that fighting it will not make it vanish.

Coping effectively with HIV is not embracing the benefits of hardship without doubt or sorrow. It is not a lighthearted acceptance of AIDS in one's life, in the gay community, in the world. It is not the ability to stay chipper in the face of great struggle. It is not simply the ability to see a profoundly important glass as half full, not half empty.

Instead, coping well with HIV is about learning to extract growth from loss. It is more about moving toward acceptance than about having reached a point of saying, "I accept this."

Such an approach makes some people anxious. Why accept what is painful, disastrous, or unfair in our life? Isn't this admitting failure?

No. Coping effectively with HIV, resurrecting a viable framework for meaning in life, involves allowing yourself to experience grievous loss along with bittersweet growth. Growth that turns a blind eye to loss is a sham. It will collapse. But loss that refuses to admit growth is no better. And the paradox of change is that something must be accepted before it can be altered.

This piece of wisdom, more than any other single coin in the treasury of psychological currency, has been crucial to the longevity and success of Alcoholics Anonymous and other self-help programs. The first key to combating alcoholism is not to fight it, but to admit it. Healing and change arise out of acceptance rather than defiance. In the long run, "I am stronger than this" proves far less effective than "I am weaker than this."

Accepting an unwanted situation or emotion, rather than fighting it, involves reorienting yourself to a different pathway of how change might come about. Our cultural notion that change is best accomplished through fighting, through strength of will—the wind blowing ever more fiercely—springs directly from our underlying assumption of personal control. Yet, as we have seen over and over, this assumption is not fact, not a universal given. It is an overblown illusion. Striving to accept our emotional stance—the sun exerting a steady presence—may in the long run achieve what fury and bustle cannot.

These, then, are ways to help build a foundation for creating an atmosphere conducive to personal change: Reaching out to others. Examining the role of control in life. Attending to pragmatic issues of health care.

Addressing (and treating) compulsive behaviors. Developing distractions. Accepting rather than fighting painful realities. These do not confer meaning to life in themselves, but they foster the right kind of climate in which growth and well-being can occur.

Although these general guidelines apply broadly, additional steps will also benefit specific individuals. In particular, let's look at how these guidelines relate to the different styles of adaptation to HIV—Transformation, Rupture, Camouflage, and Impassivity. Each suggests a somewhat different pathway for moving ahead with life's journey.

Transformation

Men who have found in HIV a catalyst for personal transformation may simply want to continue doing more of whatever they have been doing. In other words, if it ain't broke, don't fix it.

Yet even for men with this style, ongoing change and growth are still possible. Discovering meaning in life, especially in adversity, need never be a finite or static process. These men, having already met with success in integrating HIV into a new approach to life, may want to push themselves to take more risks.

Such men can be encouraged: Come out to more people as HIV-positive. Get more involved in community organizations. Go on a spiritual retreat. Become more active politically. Go back to school. Write a screenplay. Pick up the violin you haven't played in 20 years. Leave a dissatisfying relationship, or get married to your lover. The options are wide, the details less important than the overall challenge of finding new ways to continue growing.

What are the areas of life that still rankle or cause difficulty? What is an appropriate goal for continued growth? Which of my fears can I work to lessen? It is questions such as these that men with this style can use to propel them onward in further growth.

Rupture

For most men whose framework for life's meaning has been shattered by HIV, the greatest impediment to change or growth may be unresolved grief. These men must attend to the particular losses that they mourn.

Until these are healed, or in the process of healing, life will remain meaningless and bewildering.

These men experience HIV primarily as an unfair and enraging assault on their lives and the lives of those around them. They are hounded by the unanswerable question, "Why?" This question is often experienced as beyond their control—an intrusive, ruminative thought.

Yet, to the extent possible, it is helpful to find ways not to ask "Why?," to hold this question in abeyance or declare it off-limits. The more it is asked, the more damaging it becomes. There is no answer to such a question—or the answers that people find do not come by asking it. Relentlessly searching for an answer to the question of "Why?" is, yet again, responding like the wind.

Instead, the particular griefs that cause such pain, the losses that ache so sharply, must be respected, voiced, honored. And, bit by bit, worked through. Grief that feels too large or overwhelming can be addressed in small pieces, titrated into manageable doses. It may be valuable for a person to learn skills to vent some of the grief, some of the loss, without becoming overwhelmed by needing to tap into all of it at once.

In addition, a second coping strategy that may benefit men with this style begins with simply recognizing that their internal framework for life's meaning has been traumatized. In other words, it may be helpful to realize that, along with all else that has been affected, an important internal structure for coping no longer offers support. This is not an incidental occurrence, but a major psychological injury. Understanding it as such may provide new ground for regaining a sense of psychological equilibrium.

The shattering of life's meaning is an expectable response to trauma—not a desirable response, but one that can nonetheless be described, understood, and potentially healed. It is an aspect of trauma that we often feel but are unable to find words for. By calling attention to it, by naming it, we may come to find a useful new language for self-understanding, and thus begin the arduous process of building a new framework.

Camouflage

Men with the style of Camouflage are betwixt and between: fending off the despair of Rupture, but lacking the more solid foundation seen in

Transformation. Their adjustment is precarious in that it relies on half-truths and momentary spurts of enthusiasm. Unwanted information is blocked out as if it doesn't exist; painful realities or fears are superstitiously ignored. Built on shaky ground, these men's structure of meaning, and ability to cope, may crumble under pressure.

Given this situation, the most effective coping strategies for men with this style are those that bolster a person's strengths without robbing him of a needed, if imperfect, framework of beliefs. These men can benefit by scrutinizing and challenging the beliefs they hold, but gently. Which are valuable, which unrealistic or even harmful?

Such questioning may best be accomplished by discussing your ideas, fears, and hopes with other people—and being open to feedback that contradicts your expectations. A therapist, close friend, or support group can provide valuable feedback in helping fine-tune your beliefs, and in providing the safety that allows for deeper and more honest self-examination.

Getting involved in volunteer work, or some kind of altruistic behavior, may also be particularly helpful here. Such activity can provide a solid behavioral foundation to buttress shaky internal beliefs. Real-life experiences can influence the course of life's meaning; activities such as successful volunteer work can make the difference between nudging someone in the direction of Transformation or falling back into Rupture.

In addition, these are the men most prone to regard HIV as some form of punishment. Most often, this belief is unconscious but greatly influential; the idea "I deserve this" is one of the intolerable thoughts or fears a person is hiding from. It may be helpful to acknowledge and examine the influence of this belief.

Ask yourself the following questions: Do I think gay men are or were too sexually indulgent? Do I compare the relative "innocence" of various people with HIV, or various risk groups? Is it wrong for two men to have sex together? Is anal sex unnatural? If I had the choice, would I rather be straight than gay?

With a little probing, you may discover that answering "yes" to any of these questions suggests a hidden belief in HIV as punishment. Punishment for hedonism, for being sexual, for being gay. Again, this may be explicitly acknowledged or not. But to the extent that you can be open to exploring this aspect of yourself, you can then begin to try to understand and work it through. By not acknowledging that we feel punished, by not claiming this as part of our inner experience regarding AIDS, we may preclude opportunities for deeper or more substantial change—the growth that stems from facing unwanted truths rather than ignoring them.

Impassivity

In contrast to Transformation, men with a style of Impassivity may not want to change or risk too much.

For these men, stability and consistency may be the surest road to good psychological functioning. Provided that their downplaying of HIV's impact does not interfere with appropriate self-care, these men may simply want to maintain the low-key reaction that is the mainstay of their coping.

In many cases, this pattern of adaptation can be a healthy response to potential trauma. As such, these men may need to be supported in their desires not to change, not to give up their "denial," not to undergo a deep process of soul-searching. Sometimes, for some people, doing nothing *is* better than doing something.

Support for this idea comes from other research with people facing severe illness.[9] Ill people tend to develop one of two predominant coping styles in regard to their illness: vigilant focusing or minimization. Individuals who use the style of "vigilant focusing" strive to understand, manage, and track every aspect of their situation. They attempt to learn whatever they can about their illness, want exacting details about treatment options, and persistently attend to every minute facet of their medical condition. Knowledge is an anchor that keeps them moored. It is a central way of coping.

Conversely, those who minimize prefer not to know too many details. Increased knowledge may only heighten their anxiety. Too many facts, choices, and conflicting pieces of information impede their ability to cope effectively. They choose not to read what various experts say, not to learn the specifics of what may befall them, not to focus on the mountain of factual data that others so diligently seek out.

In the abstract, neither style is right, neither better than the other. Each can be adaptive or maladaptive, depending on its intensity, rigidity, and the demands of the situation. People tend to manage their anxiety best with one approach or the other. Each must be respected as a viable option— often to the chagrin or disbelief of those who rely on the opposite strategy. Again, a one-size-fits-all response does not work. What may help one person cope hinders another.

Perhaps coping with HIV, ultimately, is no more or less than the distilled essence of coping with life. Giving up the illusion of omnipotent control, forging stronger connections with other people, striving to balance fighting with acceptance—these are keys to personal growth in any situation, not just in adversity.

Yet by distilling the essence of something, don't we also change it? Living with the unwanted awareness of death's authority is certainly still living. It may even lead to richer living. But it is not the same as living with the illusion of death's nonexistence.

We tend to live, perhaps need to, with a semiconscious refusal to acknowledge that all life ends in death, that all things are impermanent. This is one of the illusions that sustains us—a fiction we eagerly mistake for fact. Life also involves suffering, and Buddhism teaches that this suffering springs directly from our unwillingness to accept the truth of impermanence.

In other words, the paradoxical key to loving life more deeply may be to relinquish our selfish investment in it.

A similar idea is expressed in Jewish mysticism. In the Kabbalah, God begins with "Nothing"—a void, an emptiness, a lack of being, beyond human contemplation.[10] But in that Nothing—embedded in it, tied to it, inseparable from it—resides everything. The Nothing never goes away. It is the same as everything. The nothingness of nonexistence and the rich full detail of life are one.

Paradox is again the key. What applies to the remote enormity of the universe applies to the irreplaceable sanctity of every life. All of us are nothing, and everything. The two are the same.

In the early days of the epidemic, I worked at Philadelphia's budding AIDS service agency—then still a small, homespun operation, penniless, disorganized; a far cry from the industry that AIDS services were soon to become. This was shortly after my friend Robby died. In no time, AIDS came to have many distinct faces, not just Robby's. I felt then, and sometimes still feel, an anger easily stoked by the irritant of governmental and societal indifference. But a deeper, more existential sense of outrage has long since waned.

What I glimpsed in that work eleven years ago was that we were unlucky enough to be living through an epidemic—*but epidemics happen all the time.* They are not new. They are not based on fairness. Somehow AIDS connected me, however fleetingly I could stay in that realm, with the universal truth of death. What hubris, that my people shouldn't die. Death awaits us all.

AIDS can trigger in us a capacity to live meaningfully, even as we live more fully knowing the deceptive illusion of our own importance. By embracing our weakness we can expand our strength. By admitting our insignificance we can know our grandeur. And by accepting the fleetingness of life, we may be open to a loving interconnection that transcends the false borders of a given moment.

Perhaps impermanence is the only truth. Need we live as if it is the only lie?

10

Grief and Hope

Columbus Day weekend, 1988, remains vivid in my memory. For the second year in a row, gay men and lesbians came together for a national march and rally in Washington, D.C. During the day the AIDS quilt lay unfurled in the nation's mall, covering acres. The quilt has an extraordinary impact, as moving in its fragility as in its size. From a distant corner of the park, a plaintive voice droned out the names of people who had died. The names blurred into one another. Most people stopped listening.

That Saturday evening, thousands of people took part in an AIDS candlelight walk and vigil. We completed the short walk in silence—a eulogy for the dead, a prayer for the living.

The evening culminated in a tepid rally. A few speakers addressed themes political and personal, but all spoke inadequately. They somehow missed the palpable, restless undercurrents of emotion in the crowd—the grief, the pride, the fear, the rage. None of the speakers came close to helping us express all that percolated beneath the surface.

The vigil ended and people milled for a few moments, awkwardly. Nobody wanted to leave, no guidance came as to how to stay. But after a few minutes, the crowd spontaneously found its voice — or voices. From one corner, a handful of people began chanting the ACT-UP slogan: "Act up! Fight back! Fight AIDS! Act up! Fight back! Fight AIDS!" With each repetition the chant grew louder. New voices joined in, new fury heated the words.

Then another chant sprang up from a different section of the crowd. It also started small, also grew more fervent with each chorus. It rang not with anger, but with solidarity: "We shall overcome, we shall overcome, we shall overcome someday, deep in my heart, I do believe we shall overcome someday. . . ."

Like magnets, each chant drew marchers to its hub. People moved spontaneously to join with one or the other. The two groups grew bigger, the chants more ardent: "Act up, fight back, fight AIDS . . . We shall overcome." Each group seemed to ignore the other, feeding off itself, drawing power or comfort from the repetitive strength of its own litany.

The chanting continued for a long time. We intoned our words to no one in particular—perhaps God, or fate, or ourselves, our private beloved specters of memory. And to the sad beauty of the candlelit night.

Perhaps relying on the rounding distortions of memory, I imbue that evening with the essence of something visceral, mythical. Some basic human stirrings found their voice: raw emotions of loss, defiant outrage at injustice, the healing anodyne of community. Yet the spontaneous outpouring seemed fueled by another, equally urgent drive—the yearning to impose some sense, some meaning, on the outrageous, the incomprehensible.

For some that night, the assault of AIDS called for defiant anger. Others felt the pain might be allayed by envisioning a future that redeemed the hardships of the present. The marchers sought out the response that best fit their temperament or current attitude. Individually, collectively, we moved toward the response that came closest to providing a sense of meaning.

I marched that evening with my then lover Kevin, and friends Jim and Matthew. Jim died in 1989, Matthew in 1993. I visited the quilt patch that day for my friend Robby, and too many others. I wonder now: How many of the marchers from that evening, whose chanting voices filled the night, are dead? How many are infected? How many have distanced themselves from AIDS, stopped caring? How many no longer fight or march or chant because the grief is just too much to bear?

How remarkable that in the face of this epidemic, we continue to carry on, to cope, to live. Some even grow and flourish. Trauma such as AIDS surely has the capacity to shatter life's meaning. Yet for many it also provides the paradoxical spark that ignites it.

This human capacity—to find meaning in even the most calamitous of events—defies easy explanation. Yet its presence must certainly be acknowledged. More than any other aspect of massive tragedy, this struggle has been evinced time and again. War, illness, natural disaster, bereavement, crippling accident, interpersonal malevolence—all lead to this quest for meaning. We strive to make sense of what befalls us, no matter how large or devastating.

Some achieve great change in facing trauma, others find relief in steadfast consistency. And perhaps a person succeeds to the degree that he or she continues to face life with courage, faith, and persistence, whatever details of meaning emerge from the struggle.

For it is meaning that people seek in times of adversity, not necessarily truth. The concept of "truth" becomes slippery here, anyway. Are the meanings that people find in trauma such as AIDS real, are they true? Do they need to be?

Some believe yes—hardship leads to truth. They see adversity as a portal into a realm of deeper truth about life. This truth may be spiritual or interpersonal. It may be about suffering or love or redemption or mettle. There are secrets about life, about the human condition, attainable only through travail.

Others, however, dismiss any such meanings as self-deception. Finding meaning in tragedy is at best a serviceable coping strategy, a clever deceit. Grasping at meaning may soothe and comfort, but it is a charade, a distorted attempt to gloss over the dismal "truth" of the situation. And that truth is of a meaningless, random, maybe even cruel, universe.

A similar dilemma often resounds through psychotherapy. Someone wonders: Is the pain I remember from my childhood "real"? Were my parents as unloving or rejecting or abusive as I recall, or do I distort the truth? What really happened?

Of course, what really happened does matter. Attempting to recreate and accept an accurate account of our experience, our truth, our past, our present, is crucial for self-understanding—in psychotherapy, with HIV, with any trauma.

But we may also speak of "emotional truth." Emotional realities warrant respect. If our emotional experience has been that of neglect, it is certainly important to try and ascertain the true extent of that neglect—but it is no less important to attend to the emotional experience of feeling neglected. That experience is also valid, regardless of the details of what happened.[1]

And so with HIV or AIDS, I do not worry too much about unanswerable questions about the "truth" of the universe. In helping people recreate new meaning in their lives in the face of HIV, I care relatively little about the deep-down reality of what is and is not true. Yes, it matters. But it is not all there is. And besides, far be it for me, or anyone, to know.

Much merit—and "truth"—lies in the quest for meaning itself. Perhaps the journey matters more than the destination. The life narratives that we weave for ourselves, our semiconscious willingness to rely on adaptive illusions, the tenacity to engage in the struggle to survive, or thrive—these are what matter. Such subjective inventions may be true or self-deceptive fancy. Either way, they are the stuff of a meaningful life.

And regardless of what is true, it is the hunger for meaning that remains constant. I am reminded of Thornton Wilder's tale, *The Bridge of San Luis Rey*. A footbridge suddenly collapses over a steep gorge, killing the five travelers who happened to be crossing at that moment. The protagonist, Brother Juniper, seeks to uncover what such a tragedy could mean—for surely it must mean something? And so he traces the lives of those who died to ascertain a meaning, the meaning for the event. Yet after carefully reconstructing the victims' lives, he is left puzzled:

> He thought he saw in the same accident the wicked visited by destruction and the good called early to Heaven. He thought he saw pride and wealth confounded as an object lesson to the world, and he thought he saw humility crowned and rewarded for the edification of the city.[2]

Where is the "truth" in the bridge's collapse? In any event of horror? In random young death, in tragedy, in the devastation of HIV? Surely it is not simply in the eye of the beholder—yet neither is it in one-size-fits-all pronouncements about the "truth" of the human condition.

Perhaps to the extent that we can struggle to balance what we know with what we hope, or stretch our tolerance for the poignant, inseparable unity of love and loss, or find nourishment enough to appease our human yearning for immortality, we can navigate adversity's shoals and find safe harbor in a life of renewed meaning.[3]

I suspect that none of the men whose lives I have depicted in these pages are all that unusual. Among people living with HIV, a few display an exceptional ability to transform their hardship into newfound vitality. Others reel from the injustice and sorrow of it. And most fall someplace in between: glimmers of growth, moments of despair, varying degrees of adaptation. For most of the men I've spoken with, HIV had ultimately neither decimated their framework of meaning, nor led to a transformative rebirth. They had adapted to living with HIV, and amid AIDS, well enough. Their style takes on the color of Transformation, Rupture, Camouflage, or Impassivity—yet it also remains anchored in constancy from who they were before.

To a large degree, perhaps most people respond to HIV as they would to any other trauma or setback—by continuing to be themselves. The fact of their infection does not alter their basic approach to life. Ultimately, their ways of coping with HIV do not deviate from their previous ways of coping. Their relative strengths and weaknesses, their general sense of self, their style of interpersonal engagement, remain the same.

Yet this is not always the case. As we have seen in a few of the men's stories, some surprise themselves, and those around them, with unprecedented transformation. Recall Stan, the unassuming bank clerk. He had never before disclosed his sexual orientation to another person, yet became a public speaker about sexuality and HIV two years into his infection. Or Francis, who, despite the fragility of his growth, had found in HIV a catalyst to finally get sober and leave a lengthy, abusive relationship. Who would have predicted either of these changes based on the evidence of their lives prior to HIV?

Unfortunately, other men also change, but not in these life-affirming ways. Their lives had seemed on course, to themselves and others, fueled by the underlying assumptions of a just, controllable, and benevolent (or at least benign) world. These assumptions had been critical to their ability to get by. Without them, their resilience crumbles. The unfairness of AIDS derails their adaptation. They become lodged in self-pity, or vitriolic anger, or passive resignation. All these are understandable, but none make for effective coping.

Why do some men adapt better than others? Why do some continue as they always have, others unravel, and others undergo transformative growth?

The best predictor of the future is the past: A person's prior style of adaptation says much about how he or she will face new stresses. But not always. Nobody can predict with certainty the routes a particular person will follow in the ongoing journey of his or her life. And I am wary of those—scientists, therapists, preachers—who claim otherwise.

Imagine how helpful it would be if we could teach someone the essence of resilience, or the keys to transformative growth. We cannot yet do so;

the alchemy involved remains mysterious. Still, much can be accomplished. We can expand our repertoire of coping strategies. We can learn new styles of social interaction and emotional expression. We can heal childhood wounds, or at least redress them to soften their pain. For most of us, it is enough to get by, and occasionally marvel at the capacity to adapt and grow, to create meaning out of chaos or sorrow.

Meaning-making is ongoing. It is a human occupation that we cannot turn off. To look at any one person in a particular moment is but an isolated snapshot that belies the fluidity of the process.

Anthony, who conveyed such wisdom and maturation when we spoke, looked much worse several years earlier. With a style more fitting Rupture than Transformation, he purposely put himself in unsafe sexual situations, potentially infecting others and raising his own risk. Likewise, it seems quite possible that Franklin, who had succeeded in getting himself off the streets, might achieve even more substantial gain if given a few more years.

Yet amid this ongoing process, a few particular events may stand out as important juncture points. One is the arrival of illness after years of outward health. The first onset of a major medical debility—the move from being HIV-positive to having AIDS—may be as powerful a disruption to psychological stability as learning that you are positive.

For some men, the growth or stability they experienced while asymptomatic crashes when they get sick. Illness becomes more than another hurdle to overcome. It derails their adaptation. For these men, as may become clear only in retrospect, their ability to get by had resided too strongly in a fantasy of personal exemption—they thought they wouldn't really get sick. This, again, is the primary risk of Camouflage. Instead of striking a balance between harsh realism and soothing illusion, such men have planted too much of their hope in the fragile soil of denial. With this gone, they have little firm ground on which to stand.

Yet the onset of illness need not be catastrophic. Despite the profound challenges posed by moving from asymptomatic to symptomatic, most men can weather this transition with the same resilience and courage that characterize other aspects of facing HIV. The arrival of illness may become but one more way station on a person's journey.

Some men experience a similar downward course over time without illness, but simply by living longer without impairment. Rather than continually gaining strength, they begin to fear that the clock is winding down.

The period of waiting becomes more onerous—is time running out? Have they beat the odds for too long?

More typically, as the years accumulate people go through phases of stability and turmoil, of optimism and hopelessness, of intrusion and denial. But to the extent that a person can still find ways to resurrect hope, or to forge a hope tempered with realism, life can continue to be a meaningful enterprise.

———————

AIDS changes rapidly. The ground keeps shifting. Medically, psychologically, demographically, much of what mattered in 1985 was antiquated by 1990. The concerns of 1996 only faintly echo those of 1991, or 2001. Moving from the individual to the communal, it strikes me that gay men are now in the midst of our third major phase of psychological reaction to living amid AIDS.

The first phase was disbelief. If you can, step back for a moment from the saturating truth of AIDS in our daily life, and you will observe something astounding: Gay men have, by and large, accommodated to AIDS' presence. We no longer express incredulity at the very fact of its existence. We take its presence for granted. It is horrible and unwanted, a source of scabrous misery. Yet it no longer offends our basic view of reality: AIDS is part of reality.

Over the years we have moved from disbelief—"This cannot be"—to incorporating the fact of AIDS into our expectations about life. How extraordinary the ability, given time, to acclimate to something even so incomprehensible as an epidemic! We abhor AIDS and are outraged by it, but we no longer say to ourselves, "This cannot be."

A reaction of disbelief was most prominent in the early years of the epidemic. The second major phase, overlapping with the first but then supplanting it, was action.

AIDS descended with the fury of a whirlwind. Much needed to be done. While not quite taking in the full brunt of what lay ahead, gay men responded with a stamina and maturity that had not previously characterized our communities. In very little time, gay men formed social service agencies to offer care, support, and education. Clever, effective safe-sex campaigns were conceived and launched. A slew of activist organizations sprang up, most prominently ACT-UP. Newsletters, underground drug networks, community-based drug trials, theater groups, lobbying organizations—an entire new subculture, the "AIDS world," developed in the span of a few brief years. A wide range of active responses emerged to meet the crisis before us.

Much of the action was effective, some was not. Yet regardless of what worked and what didn't, the fact of so much action is significant in itself. Perhaps the unconscious motto of coping with AIDS for many years was "Do Something." It didn't matter what: volunteer work, fundraising, activism, lobbying, civil disobedience, whatever. Just do *something*.

Clearly, much needed (and still needs) to be done—but this was not all that drove the intensity of action. Action fueled a sense of optimism that the epidemic could be ameliorated. It combated the helplessness that arises when faced with overpowering external forces. It reinvigorated a belief in personal control over what seemed uncontrollable. The response of action was borne from an attempt to maintain life's meaning: The driving unconscious hope was that AIDS could be tamed or destroyed through the channels people had previously relied on to overcome obstacles.

While many results of this period of action were of great value, individually and collectively, the response of action cannot help but to have failed in its unconscious wish. It has not stopped the dying. Hope that action could restore life's meaning has been sorely tested; for many this belief has been completely nullified. And so we are no longer in a time of action.

We now face the third phase of life with AIDS—the burden of cumulative grief. What I see as "grief-overload" is the defining and most prominent emotional feature on the landscape today. It is the most dangerous psychological realm that we have entered.

More than anything else, this central fact of modern gay life must be acknowledged: Ours has become an age, a culture, of grief. Most of this grief is hidden, unexpressed. But it powerfully influences our current behavior, and future adaptation, in what continues to be an ongoing crisis.

Perhaps it is not possible for individuals, or a community, to sustain an acute level of emotion over too long a time. We cannot keep crying, keep raging, keep aching, keep fighting, keep caring. After a certain point exhaustion wins out. The acuity of pain corrodes into numbness. The cumulative disappointments of failed action make it difficult to spark yet another new assault.

Grief has many textures. Collectively, our grief is no longer—or not currently—a sharp keening. It is a grief of fatigue and defeat. We are in the midst of grief too powerful to assimilate, too unwieldy to mourn. It is expressed more through apathy than tears, more through withdrawal than engagement. We are numb with loss.

But this is still grief, and we must try to see it as such.

AIDS no longer grabs headlines, no longer causes a sensation. It has become just one more of life's difficulties, one more media horror competing for our attention. It is no longer fashionable. Fewer celebrities wear red ribbons at the Oscars.

It would be easy to blame this growing indifference toward AIDS on the homophobic antipathy of straight society. That certainly may be a factor, yet such an explanation is incomplete. The indifference rings true in the gay world as well: AIDS seldom makes headline news even in the gay press. It receives decreasing, and less urgent, attention. We have moved beyond a time of focused awareness into something much harder to fight.

Our distance from AIDS hit home for me at the closing ceremonies of the Gay Games IV at Yankee Stadium in New York in June 1994, part of the twenty-fifth commemoration of the Stonewall Riots. The stadium was sold out—Yankee Stadium sold out for a gay cultural event! It seemed a monumental achievement, a milestone. Surely this indication of how far we have come in the struggle to claim the regularity of our lives is an event of major societal impact.

Amid all the hoopla, the speeches, the performances, the dedications, the parade of athletes, no moment was set aside to remember our dead, our dying, our ill, our caregivers. AIDS was not present. It was as if AIDS did not exist, or was not to be mentioned lest it spoil the fun. As if it were not an omnipresent reality. Would such an omission have occurred a few years prior?

Ron provided a vivid description of the difficulty of living amid the constant awareness of AIDS' impact:

> [It's like] being on the scene of a bad auto accident. You're struck by
> the tragedy of it, but you have to pick up the dry cleaning, or there's
> a meeting you've got to attend.

To the extent possible, we need to remind ourselves that we live with an ever-present car accident. We need to remind ourselves that the crisis is not over, that the infections and illness and dying and need for optimism have

not stopped. We need to do this not to revel in pain, not to flagellate ourselves with guilt. But to know the extent of our losses so that we may continue to live. And to reach out and care for our young: We must face our
grief to help them face theirs.

For perhaps the most disturbing trend of the past few years has been
the unexpected increase in HIV rates among gay men, and particularly
young gay men. The safer-sex initiatives of the 1980s no longer work. For
years, gay men succeeded in adopting new sexual styles — a move once
hailed as "the most profound modification of personal health-related
behaviors ever recorded."[4] But this is no longer the case. We now witness new waves of infection among men who know how to behave safely
but do not.

And perhaps more than anything else, this trend relates to the enormity,
and hiddenness, of our grief. Grief in the guise of "Why bother?" Grief in
the mistaken idea that becoming infected is inevitable. Grief in the bot-
tomless, empty feeling of "I've lost too much anyway."

What has led to this overload? More than anything else is the human
difficulty of sustaining any strong emotion at too high a pitch. Perhaps this
is the primary reason for the fading of AIDS from our daily awareness, for
the move from fervor and action to weariness and disengagement.

Yet other factors are also relevant. One is the sad fact of AIDS' stub-
born ability to outwit medicine. Our science is not yet a match for it. Several years of heady discoveries—the isolation of HIV, the development of
antibody screening assays, AZT and other antiviral and prophylactic treatments — gave way to an extended period of relative quiescence on the
medical front. Improvements continually chip away at some of the grim-
mer aspects of AIDS, and life expectancies continually improve; recent
developments even suggest a long-awaited period of substantial progress.
But chipping only does so much. For too long, science has been unable to
rekindle the emotional energy needed to reverse the apathy that weighs us
down.

And too many of us have died. Beyond the grief is the fact of so many
actual lives lost. Too many of our leaders, our protesters, our doctors, our
artists, our compatriots, our lovers, are dying or dead. Too many expressions of rage, of anguish, of cogent activism, have been silenced. Too many
unknown voices have left us without ever being heard.

Death counts are more than an abstraction. They have taken their toll.
The number of dead is great enough so that the absence of an entire cadre
of men can be felt—for those who can bear to feel it.

The AIDS apathy and burnout that characterize the current years, the diminution of ACT-UP and activism, the soaring rate of new infections among young gay men, the nihilistic, self-destructive abandonment of safer-sex practices because "we're all going to die anyway"—all these relate to an inability to grieve. As a community, we are clogged with a grief that goes unexpressed and dampens our ability to live. And depending on how we meet the psychological challenges we now face, several possibilities lie in store for what is to come.

Until we can discover ways to bear and express our losses, the numbness that characterizes this current phase will continue. What can help us out of this straightjacket?

A medical breakthrough may play a pivotal role in resurrecting hope, ushering in a period of renewed energy and commitment. Yet depending on what that breakthrough may be, this spark may have potentially unwanted results.

For example, if current progress in hampering the virus also results in a vaccine to halt new infections, this will surely be a joyous accomplishment. But it will have complicated effects on our communities. It may help bridge a division between positive and negative men, taking away the risks of sex. But it also may further isolate HIV-positive men, creating a marked bloc of people who are to be AIDS' last targets.

Medical progress, of some nature or other, will surely arrive. But this alone will not propel us beyond our grief, nor can we count on it.

We need onion cellars.

In his novel *The Tin Drum*, Gunter Grass evokes a surreal, burlesque world to capture the experience of World War II in Germany. In the years following the war, after Germany begins to regain a sense of social and economic stability, Grass tells of a fictitious cosmopolitan nightclub, the Onion Cellar.

The Onion Cellar is an unusual place. It serves no food or drink, offers no conventional entertainment. Instead, well-heeled patrons sit at crude tables, where they are given cutting boards, paring knives, and onions. They wait obediently until the club owner instructs them to cut and peel the onions. They start timidly. But then they cut and peel with abandon.

And they begin to cry. Their crying soon turns to wailing, a communal grief mirrored in a skein of individual tears. The patrons turn to their friends and to strangers, weeping and comforting each other. They confess their sins, their hurts, their guilt. They use the onions to gain access to the pain they carry but cannot otherwise express. They come to the Onion Cellar to share this pain publicly, because the experience is less fulfilling if one cuts onion at home and cries alone. Some patrons come only once, others repeatedly, until exhausted of their tears. And somehow, in the process, they feel healed.

This is what we face with AIDS right now. We need onion cellars. As a community, as shared witnesses and bearers of so much loss, we must find ways to express the pain, the grief, the despair that feels increasingly out of our scope—and to do so safely, emotionally, repeatedly. And we must do so communally, so that others may be there as support and witness, so that we may all serve as comforter and mourner.

The AIDS quilt has served such a function. Its ability to provide this kind of communal memorial underlies its power. Perhaps more than any other undertaking, it has been our onion cellar. But other avenues are needed as well. We need to claim our grief.

Some ways to do this may be easily within our grasp, and others require forging new rituals. We need community-based memorial services. Grief workshops. Theater performances, art, dance, sculpture, music. Days of mourning. Rituals and commemorations to fit the needs of a new reality.

One such possible ritual is an African tradition, the Calling of Names. For the past several years, the Outwrite conference (an annual gathering of gay and lesbian writers) has opened with this invocation. As the conference begins, the amassed group of participants are invited to reflect on those who have died, and to call their names out loud so that they may join us. The tradition is based in the belief that as long as a person is remembered, he or she continues to be part of the communal life, the collective immortality. The Calling of Names is done so that people will not be forgotten. And it is a way to mark and respect our own grief, while continuing on with life.

Perhaps more than anything else, we must begin again simply to address the topic. Acknowledging that we grieve is a crucial step in grieving. Our ongoing struggle with HIV—the continued triumphs, the continued tragedy—must be named, spoken, written of, reclaimed as a prime focus of attention.

And to the extent possible, we must try to fight against a process that grows ever more pronounced: a division between gay men who are HIV-positive and HIV-negative.

Ironically, this distinction between positive and negative men grew out of an important medical advance: the widespread acceptance of antibody testing. Until this process became routine in the late 1980s, uncertainty regarding infection encouraged a kinship among all those who might be at risk. Within the gay community, antibody testing gained favor (after years of heated controversy) because of its potential health benefits. Yet being able to know our HIV status has created a different track for those with and without the virus.

For many gay men—positive and negative, each for different reasons— the presence or absence of HIV provides a rationale for making an "us versus them" distinction. Those living with HIV may feel that HIV-negative men shun them, or cannot understand their experience, or that negative men have been unfairly let off the hook because their mortality is not at stake. For men who are negative, the division stems from fear, relief, survivor guilt, and the withdrawal (often unconscious) from association with something life-threatening.

To ignore the psychological concerns of HIV-negative men is mistaken. In the quake of any catastrophe, would we want to disregard the pain of those who witnessed and felt the trauma, who bore immense grief, but who happened to survive? In the family of an ill person, would we ever assume that the only person affected by the illness was the patient?

Yet the reality of AIDS is also that HIV-positive men have unique and greater stresses to bear. Most fundamental, of course, is the fact of mortality. When the basic threat to your existence is gone, as it is for HIV-negative men who continue to act safely, the challenges to be faced are of a whole different sort.

It is misleading, and potentially harmful, to cast a distinction between HIV-positive and HIV-negative men too sharply. Who, after all, are the men making up the new waves of seroconversion? How many men who think themselves negative do so based on the faded assurance of an old antibody test? Being HIV-negative is determined by what we do, not who we are. A danger of being HIV-negative is to treat the news as a stable personality trait—or to act as such.

Perhaps having some sort of "us versus them" view is unavoidable for most people, an artifact of our basic tendency to categorize and sort information, to organize the world. Ironically, it may even spring from beneficial motives. Perhaps the root of prejudice is not hate, but short-sighted love—

the desire to protect the kinships and communities that matter the most to us, to strengthen the bonds with those with whom we feel closest.[5] But where one draws the line between who is "us" and who is "them" is movable, with important consequences.

I lead a psychotherapy group for gay men. In the group, one of the members frequently discusses feeling isolated and different from the other men, a sense of alienation within the group that mirrors his life outside. He speaks of a wall that separates him from all the other members. He feels this wall almost as a literal presence in the room, one that safely encloses the other members but excludes him.

In a simple move with significant repercussions, another group member finally suggested that such a wall did exist—but argued that it enclosed the entire group, not just select members. The wall separated those within the room from those outside it. It encircled the whole group, and all within were included, all as gay men. Perhaps for the first time in his adult life, the first group member began to feel that he was part of something, that he belonged. And even though the wall was recast around the room, this led to his feeling more of a sense of belonging outside the group as well.

We can all build walls in a range of places. We need not base it on the presence or absence of HIV.

In introducing this book I presented myself as a researcher, a psychotherapist, and a gay man. I am also HIV-negative. To start the work as such felt too awkward an introduction. (Was this an expression of my guilt, my shame, my concern that my words would be disqualified?) To close by saying nothing feels dishonest. And so I choose to disclose my status here, in the specific context of expressing concern over the harmful division between positive and negative gay men.

To help us (all of us) overcome our grief, to help us return to more vital living amid a world of loss, to help welcome young gay men into a safe and diverse community, we must work against this distinction. Let us keep an "us versus them" worldview if we need to. Many real-life "thems" exist for us to rally and fight against. But let us not divide from within our own ranks. Let us not split our own home.

What will happen when AIDS, as we know it, ends? When a vaccine arrives, when medical progress robs AIDS of its lethality, or when a cure destroys the virus? In the aftermath of any major development that curtails AIDS' presence in our lives, I believe that gay men can anticipate some sort of communal post-traumatic stress reaction.

During a crisis, people typically suppress their emotions to function effectively. It is when the threat recedes that deeper feelings emerge, and must be reckoned with. The same holds true, in large part, with an ongoing trauma such as AIDS: Even with the burden of grief that colors the day, we are still in crisis mode. The actual depth of our anguish has not yet been voiced.

The history of trauma—large, small, communal, individual—tells us over and over that psychological reactions do not stop when a trauma ends. The residue may linger for years to come. Holocaust survivors did not simply forget Nazi barbarism after liberation. War veterans do not leave behind their harsh memories when they quit the battlefield. Individuals whose loved ones die in sudden or shocking ways often feel plagued years later with depression and the continued inability to find meaning in life.

The sorrow that goes unexpressed now — because it is too much, because it interferes with the more pressing task of caring for the ill—will have its due. If not now, later. For those living through the epidemic and immersed in it, AIDS will not stop when it stops.

To some extent, such a post-traumatic reaction may be unavoidable. Yet lessons from other traumas also tell us that it can be tempered if we attend now to the pain we suppress.

The concept of "anticipatory grief" is relevant here. Individuals who have time to prepare for the loss of a loved one, who can begin their grieving process before the actual death, typically fare better in the long run than those who have no such opportunity. Having time to prepare, to experience some of the emotions of loss, to say "goodbye" or "I love you" or whatever else needs be said, minimize the likelihood of a prolonged grief reaction. In the short term it may feel no different—the loss still registers heavily. But the long haul is eased.

And so again I return to the importance of finding ways to voice our grief. Not only to rediscover a sense of energy to fuel our lives, but to lessen the load for what we may need to face in the years to come.

Several years have passed since I conducted the interviews that appear in these pages. Now, as I reflect on the paths of meaning offered in these pages—the ten representations, the four styles—I sometimes find myself floating adrift in the intermingling currents of individual and community. Each of us exists as a world unto himself. Each of us also exists as part of something larger. We are all part and whole simultaneously.

Perhaps the responses that seem so pronounced in certain people are only facets of a larger organismic response. A community or society, no matter how disorganized or amorphous, can be thought of as one organism, one living entity, one body.

Each of the men I spoke with had a distinct reaction to HIV and AIDS. Kyle tasted its bitterness firsthand when his lover died, but then accomplished tremendous personal growth. Ron sank into a world of bewilderment and grief. Craig mustered a feisty arrogance that stretched credible boundaries of denial but helped inoculate him against despair and terror.

Viewed differently, each merely carried some portion of a more encompassing response to massive trauma—as do we all. The growth, the grief, the struggle, the triumph, the fear, the resignation—individually, we differ in emphasis. Together, we each hold a fragment of the greater yearning to seek meaning in events that exceed our ken.

And we are all part of something beyond ourselves. Early on, in AIDS' first few agonizing years of disbelief and sharp grief, I remember taking peculiar solace in knowing that AIDS would not end homosexuality. Looking back now with a language I lacked then, I see how this was crucial in my own struggle to maintain life's meaning in the crisis: finding purpose in belonging, deriving comfort in the idea of symbolic immortality. AIDS would take many of us; we were on the cusp of what seemed destined to mount into warlike bereavement. Many of us would live, many would die. But no matter its toll, AIDS would not destroy homosexuality. That would endure. Time, nature, and procreation would see to that.

Given the particularity of how our lives crossed, each of the men from the study was invited to stay in touch with me, but only if he so chose. I am grateful that several have done so. Some, I know, have died. Others are living with AIDS, with varying degrees of impairment. A few others, to quote Anthony, are "just HIV and doing pretty well."

Ron called me one year after our interview. He asked if we could meet again. When we got together this second time, he looked much more frail.

He seemed not far from death, with that indescribable AIDS visage that replaces the rich individuality of a healthy face. Yet he also seemed more energetic.

We spoke for an hour or two. He recalled our first meeting in detail, and was not surprised at my assessment that AIDS had shattered his life's meaning. But in the intervening year, even as his body had deteriorated, his inner torment had lessened. He had made some peace with the demons that had plagued him before. He thought himself wiser, calmer. His grief over his lost lover Robert remained strong. It was less sharp than it had been, but still the emotional brunt of his life.

I asked why he wanted to meet again. He said he would like a transcript of our interview to use in planning his memorial service. He thought our talk offered the most complete testament available of his inner thoughts and feelings; he wanted to send copies to two close friends and his minister.

Ron had other reasons for wanting to meet as well. After speaking briefly, he took out a photo album he had brought along. He called it "the family album." It was an antique green scrapbook, caringly assembled with pictures of him, Robert, a few former lovers and friends, the men from his one-time communal household. He had put the album together only recently, as memorial, anthology, and wish. Oh, the wish! The last page was a glistening, youthful picture of he and Robert in each other's arms, smiling, carefree. Eons had passed since the picture was taken; perhaps five years. He said he often dreamt of that picture. He hoped that was what awaited him after death.

A few weeks later he sent me a poem he had written:

Autumn 1991

I have begun
to look like Lincoln
in the last year
of his life,
bony and gaunt.
Those great sad eyes
sunk in their sockets,
hair a haystack tumble.
The war finally won

the battle most surely
lost.

O Robert, we may soon
be together,
but how I will miss
this sweet struggle,
ever the rebel.

Open your arms.
I come to you
for our rocking,
nevermind the repose.
We'll make those
heavenly bedsprings moan.

During this second meeting, Ron asked that in my book, I not protect his confidentiality, that I not present him anonymously. He wanted to be identified by his name, with his life. He said: "These things happened and I feel no embarrassment about them. I need no anonymity."

By bringing me his family album, by asking that he be remembered by name, I believe Ron hoped I might serve as a vessel to help keep him alive. This, as much as collecting the transcript, seemed his purpose in reconnecting. Our meetings had become more than an incidental detour in his journey of living and dying. They had entered into his stream of meaning-making. Ron came to see his participation in this project, and the possibility of his words being available to others, as a tool to help him create meaning: belonging, continuity, altruism, memorial, symbolic immortality.

Ron Woolson died in January 1993. I hope I have honored his wishes with an accurate portrayal of his struggles and triumphs.

Lucas also contacted me, several years after our first meeting. The growth and resilience he had demonstrated in our first encounter seemed even more impressive.

Lucas had given up the pulpit years earlier, soon after learning of his infection. But the minister in him was never far from the surface, even in our individual meetings. He spoke with a powerful, majestic presence.

Poetry was of great importance to him, and he ably communicated the emotional depth and complexity of the poems that mattered to him.

In the course of our several meetings, Lucas has read me several poems. He has a particular and rather endearing habit — quite ministerial — of reciting each poem twice, presumably to allow the deeper meanings of the poem to unfold with repetition. They usually do.

In our first interview, the poems Lucas chose all spoke to the frightening uncertainty of dying and death, the meaningless of life. Despite his predominantly growth-oriented spiritual response to HIV, there was also a strong undercurrent of questioning his faith: "I don't understand why, HIV now in my life. God and I have a lot of knock-down, drag-out fights about this one, because I can't see it." Four years later, however, the poems and readings that Lucas shares with me are of a different nature. He no longer struggles with the "why" of his infection. He feels more secure in his acceptance of the cycle of living and dying, of tragedy and growth inseparable.

Lucas has come out as HIV-positive to most of his family and friends. He believes his relationship with his lover Douglas, who has remained negative, is stronger than ever; the two recently marked their twentieth anniversary with a large celebration. He chose not long ago to discontinue treatment with AZT, based on his concern about its adverse effects. His T-cell count has since climbed by 100.

The last time we met, Lucas once again ended with a quote, appropriately ministerial, from a homily preached at an AIDS healing service at a church in Boston:

> The miracle of Love rises from the ashes of our broken dreams;
> The light of hope is kindled in the shadows of our unspeakable loss.[6]

Lucas is often present in my thoughts, my prayers, my work as a psychotherapist. So are the other men. In a way I can't quite describe, but as an honor I accept, a part of them has become a part of me.

Epilogue

The Current Moment

July, 1996

$\mathcal{T}$he 11th International Conference on AIDS, held in Vancouver, nears an end. Unlike previous conferences, this one shimmers with barely restrained optimism. Headlines once again overflow with news of HIV. Words once unthinkable—management, containment, cure—suddenly suffuse the austere language of professional dialogue and the eager, fingers-crossed, "dare I hope?" conversations and prayers of those whose lives are most affected. As this book goes to press, we may be witnessing a much-awaited turning point in our long, wearying battle.

It is premature to determine whether the optimism that shapes current discussion is a bubble soon to burst, or the beginning of a new, and maybe even closing, chapter in defeating the virus. We can only hope that the new drug therapies will realize and sustain their tantalizing promise.

While believing (and hoping) that we may indeed be rounding a crucial corner, I also cannot help but see the unbridling of such optimism as a counterpoint to the energy-sapping pessimism of the past several years. That pessimism was paralyzing, and only partly deserved—we have been steadily gaining ground all along. But the optimism that now carries the day may also be too strong. Perhaps it is our understandable yearning for such optimism, for good news, that fuels the sudden turnabout, as

227

much as the facts before us? This is the first hook we have long had on which to hang our hopes. Our hopes may be stronger than any hook can realistically hold.

None of the recent advances, or the unknown others that will no doubt follow, diminish our ongoing need to cope with the crisis. But the context changes. Substantial medical progress will usher in a new phase of personal and communal psychological reaction to HIV. This may be the trigger needed to catapult us beyond the numbness that has leeched our vitality over the past several years. And if the progress is true, we must also expect a launch into the more acute work of grief that still beckons unattended. The joy of any triumphant medical advance will be intertwined with releasing the pain and disbelief we carry from too many years of astounding loss.

Last week, a patient told me of an acquaintance's death. This did not shock him; he had already experienced many other deaths, and regarded them as an unhappy but expectable commonplace. Such are our lives. But he noted, with irony, a somewhat different reaction to hearing of this one. It seemed harder to tolerate, sadder, and more outrageous, when viewed against the backdrop of the changing news. In some ways now, how much more challenging and difficult the ambiguities of life with HIV may be— how much more bewildering and maddening that people are still getting sick, still succumbing, still dying.

Our current dilemma can be likened to a decisive battle in the midst of a long war. At a certain point, one may glimpse that the direction of a war's outcome is becoming more clear—victory, long hoped-for, begins to seem realistic or probable. But it is not victory yet. Many a skirmish remain to be fought. Planning strategies, maintaining faith and constancy, continuing to gear up for battle in one's personal tried-and-true manner, become no less urgent. And many lives will still be lost.

We may, finally, be nearing such a moment. But much looms ahead. The crisis is not over, medically or psychologically. Not for those facing a mountain of bereavement. Not for those infected individuals fortunate enough to be well-insured, savvy health-care consumers. And certainly not for the majority of those affected in America and throughout the world.

The face of AIDS is changing. The challenges to life's meaning remain with us, influenced, but by no means erased, by where science leads us today and tomorrow. AIDS' impact will reach far beyond the taming of HIV.

Yet how sweet the fantasy I can now briefly allow myself to indulge, imagining a day when this book, this chronicle of a community drenched in loss, will be an antiquated document of a time gone by.

I dreamed

I dreamed everyone
came back. Some

chose to return
healthy, one had to

exercise memory
to remind of name;

some came back with
marks of illness, stamped

by disease's design.
Everyone was applauded,

appreciated, re-
acclimated. It was,

after all, a miracle.
It was, after all,

a dream.

Walta Borawski

Appendix A

The Men in the Study

Anthony: Anthony held a Master's degree in Library Sciences, specializing in old and rare manuscripts. At 39, he had known of his immune impairment for nine years—longer than any of the other men in the study, and prior to the actual discovery of HIV. Despite the many friends who had died, and occasional health impairments, he continued to live a full life, including a new job and new relationship. Alcoholics Anonymous (AA) philosophy and Roman Catholicism were central to his worldview.

Charles: At 39, Charles had known his HIV status for three years, and had expected a positive test result before that. He met his current lover in an HIV support group. Involved with Alcoholics Anonymous, Narcotics Anonymous, and Sex and Love Addicts Anonymous, Charles said of his HIV infection, "It feels like just another meeting for me." The death of a close friend one month ago before we met left him overcome with grief and fears about the future.

Craig: 30 years old, Craig tested positive 18 months prior to our meeting; it confirmed what he had already assumed: His two previous lovers had both died of AIDS, and the test result was simply "gilding the lily." Proudly gay-identified and committed to social change, Craig regarded HIV as a "nuisance" that interfered with his life. His health had not been affected by HIV. While he worries vaguely about the future, his current low-key reaction to his infection was summed up in his belief, "If I feel fine, I'm fine."

Eugene: A 46-year-old "community organizer," Eugene had led an un-conventional, somewhat bohemian life, pursuing various artistic endeavors and working as a grassroots political organizer for different progressive causes. His positive test result, four years before our interview, came as a great shock. Eugene used activity as a primary way of coping with HIV: He is extremely involved in the social and community politics of HIV and AIDS.

Francis: At 42, Francis had gone through profound changes in the six years of knowing he was HIV-positive: He kicked a severe alcohol habit that he believes would have killed him, and he finally left a long-standing, emotionally abusive relationship. His sense of rebirth was such that he thought of throwing himself a "six-year-old birthday party" to mark the date of his positive test. Devoutly religious, he told me with unadorned conviction, "HIV is my blessing."

Franklin: In some ways, this 31-year-old African-American man experi-enced more dramatic HIV-triggered life changes than any other study par-ticipant. He was a severe alcoholic, and HIV had led him, over the past two years, first to sobriety, then to the beginning of a life off the streets and out of the shelters of Philadelphia. He now goes into inner city neighborhoods to share his story and talk about AIDS. But his process of growth remains incomplete: He still engages in unsafe sex, and routinely skips medical appointments if he fears something is wrong.

Harris: 37 years old, Harris had known about his HIV status for approximately 5 years. An affable, intelligent, extremely self-deprecating man, Harris had something about him of the cartoon character "Richie Rich: Poor Little Rich Boy." He came from a privileged background and lived in an apartment crammed with magnificent art, but had never held a challenging job or found a fulfilling adult avocation. HIV had neither hindered nor facilitated a search for meaning in Harris' life: It seemed of secondary importance compared to whatever factors kept him unfulfilled in the first place.

Howard: A 45-year-old academically respected art historian, Howard lived and taught in New York City. He learned he was HIV-positive when his lover, Seth, was diagnosed with AIDS in 1985. Seth died in 1987.

Moderately secretive about his homosexuality and extremely secretive about his HIV-infection, Howard had not experienced any health difficulties. But as a gay black male academic professional, Howard felt little sense of connection or similarity with the other people in his world.

Jules: A shy, likeable, introverted 27-year-old man, Jules was infected at the age of 19 in his first sexual experience, when he was taken advantage of by two older men. He had confided his HIV status to very few other people, but recently told his parents. He felt alienated from other HIV-positive men, in large part because he was never "promiscuous" and didn't want to be thought of as such.

Kyle: A 45-year-old former high school teacher, Kyle was employed in an AIDS service organization when we met. He had known about his status since his lover, Frank, was diagnosed only days before his death in 1985. Frank was Kyle's first male lover; he had been married for many years, with one teenage son. Despite his report of occasional debilities, Kyle radiated a sense of health. HIV had initiated tremendous growth in his life.

Leon: A 35-year-old physician, Leon's "whole world just fell apart" when he learned he was positive two years before we met—and weeks before his graduation from medical school. Living for many years in a monogamous relationship with his partner (who was HIV-negative), Leon had not had high risk sex since 1981. For Leon, living with HIV has been a profound, bittersweet experience: He has come to "treasure" life and his relationship, but he is also painfully fearful of imminent loss. AIDS is everpresent in his thoughts. He believes HIV has made him a more compassionate doctor.

Lucas: At 40, Lucas is a minister and therapist with a doctorate in pastoral counseling. After learning he was positive two years before we met, he was tremendously relieved to learn he had not transmitted HIV to his lover of 15 years. Bolstered by his strong religious beliefs, keen intellect, and his lover's support, Lucas actively struggles to use his HIV infection as a catalyst for a fuller life.

Nate: 46 years old. A financially successful businessman, Nate abruptly retired when he received his unexpected positive test result 34 months before we met. He assumed he would only be alive for a couple of years; still healthy, he's running out of money. In his search to spend his time meaningfully, Nate volunteers a great deal of time and energy for an AIDS service organization. Yet he is dismayed that, at his age and in his situation, he still lacks a sense of purpose or fulfillment in life.

Ron:　Ron looked older than his 44 years, due to HIV-related intestinal difficulties, general weight loss, and unresolved grief for his lost lover, Robert, who died the year before we met. He had known of his infection for five years, when a former boyfriend died. He left his job one year earlier, after fatigue and memory impairments affected his ability to work. The pain of his many losses was apparent in our meeting, as was his rage and bewilderment at how AIDS "steals the time that was rightfully ours."

Sam:　At 50, Sam came to discover his homosexuality relatively late in life. After he was divorced in his late thirties, a girlfriend introduced him to "swinging." He found that he preferred male partners to female, and began avidly pursuing gay sexual encounters. He tested HIV-positive in 1985. His lover of four years has AIDS. In the past several years he had revealed—with great relief—his homosexuality and his HIV status to his extended family, his children, and his co-workers in the construction firm where he had worked for 25 years.

Stan:　A 48-year-old bank clerk who tested HIV-positive 18 months before we met, Stan had assumed he was HIV-positive. A recent bout of pancreatitis, triggered by a bad reaction to an experimental drug, resulted in weight loss and hospitalization. A quiet man who had never had an intimate relationship or acknowledged his homosexuality to friends, co-workers, or family, HIV has led to a newfound sense of openness and belonging to the gay community.

Victor:　At 42, Victor had spent years revelling in the sexual saturnalia of Manhattan's cutting edge gay life—and he has "no regrets, period." He wasn't surprised when he tested positive in the late 1980s; most of his friends and his long-term lover were already dead. Weakened now by fatigue and weary of so much continually mounting grief, he contemplates suicide. But a passionate, rebellious anger and a sharply acerbic wit suggest that much life struggles within him yet, despite his depression.

Vincent: At 27 and one of the youngest men in the study, Vincent was also the most robustly optimistic. With the effervescence and enthusiasm of a one man Chamber of Commerce, his likeable, glib manner suggested a deep (and useful) belief in the power of positive thinking. Vincent had known he was positive for 17 months. He had experienced no health impairments, and had had no contact with people with AIDS.

Willy: A 34-year-old professional waiter, Willy tested positive 27 months before we met. Weight loss and fatigue had affected his daily functioning. He had never had a lover or boyfriend. A close friend, whom he nursed through illness, died several months before we met. A gentle, gracious, and lonely man, Willy struggled to get on with life and keep the despair he clearly felt as far away as possible.

Appendix B

Research Data

Background

In 1990–1991, I conducted this study as part of my doctoral training in clinical psychology. My general aim was to learn more about the impact of HIV and AIDS on life's meaning. The research was guided by the following questions: (1) How, if at all, have HIV-positive gay men found meaning in, or made sense of, AIDS? (2) What are the strategies HIV-positive gay men use to maintain or reconstitute the belief in a meaningful world? (3) How has AIDS affected beliefs about such issues as fate, religion, death, the meaning or purpose of life, and the degree to which people control their own destiny?

The study had broad theoretical underpinnings in the humanist-existentialist psychological literature on "massive death" experiences (e.g. Dimsdale, 1980; Frankl, 1959; Lifton, 1980). A basic thread running through this literature is that survivors of great trauma need to establish some meaning or purpose in the profoundly disrupting events that jar their lives. More narrowly, the study was informed by a cognitive perspective on trauma, and especially Assumptive World theory (Janoff-Bulman, 1992). According to this theory, people rely on several core assumptions about themselves and the world, usually held unconsciously. Trauma's greatest potential harm may result from the shattering or nullifying of these basic, underlying assumptions—and the challenge of recovery is reestablishing a set of beliefs that can once again provide meaning, self-esteem, and coherence.

Subjects

Participants in the study were 19 HIV-positive gay men, none of whom met diagnostic criteria for AIDS, as then defined by the Centers for Disease Control (1987). All participants had known of their seropositivity for at least 18 months, so none of the men were reacting to an initial phase of "shock." Nine of the men had never experienced any HIV-related health impairment. Six had experienced minor symptoms, and four had experienced more significant difficulties, including weight loss and continual fatigue. None had a history of major health difficulty prior to HIV infection.

Sixteen of the men were white, two African-American, and one Latino. They ranged in age from 27 to 50 years old, with a median age of 40 and a mean age of 39. They had known about their HIV status for between 18 and 106 months (median: 34 months; mean: 41 months; one participant [Anthony] knew of his impairment before the discovery of HIV). All but one of the participants (Franklin) were economically stable. The men were well educated: seven had a postgraduate degree, another seven had graduated from college, and four of the remaining five had some college education. All lived in urban settings with well established gay communities.

Subjects were recruited by three methods: word of mouth, a flyer describing the study, and a brief description of the study offered by the researcher at HIV-related community events.

Procedure

Given its exploratory nature, the study employed a qualitative, phenomenological research design (Polkinghorne, 1989). The primary tool of the study was an intensive semi-structured interview. Data were analyzed *post hoc*, rather than with *a priori* assumptions or hypotheses.

Each subject participated in a lengthy, individual, semi-structured clinical interview. Participants were told prior to the interview that the general aim of the study was to learn about their experiences, attitudes, and thoughts regarding their current life situation. Interviews included the following general categories of information: gay self-identity; relationships; HIV-related changes in sexual behaviors and attitudes; general psychosocial adaptation to HIV; issues of mortality, death, and illness; current medical concerns and treatment approaches; experiences with grief and bereavement; thoughts about AIDS in the gay community; spirituality; and substance abuse.

Interview questions were determined beforehand by the researcher, along with two other psychologists and a microbiologist with expertise in AIDS research. Two pilot interviews were conducted (included among the 19), during which specific interview questions were honed and finalized. All interviews were conducted by the researcher. The researcher had prior experience working with HIV issues in professional and volunteer settings.

The interviews followed a semi-structured format, in that particular questions and topics remained consistent from subject to subject, but followed the individualized conversational flow of the specific interview. Great emphasis was placed on establishing rapport between the researcher and participant.

Each participant was interviewed once. The interviews lasted between 90 minutes and three hours, with the majority taking approximately two and one-half hours. In all situations, the interview occurred in a private setting. All interviews were audiotaped and then transcribed verbatim. Participants were invited to remain in contact with the researcher; several chose to do so. The interviews took place between November 1990 and April 1991.

Data Analysis

Data analysis involved two phases. The goal of the first phase was to determine the specific qualities, traits, "meaning units" (Giorgi, 1985), or connotations the men attributed to AIDS and HIV. This phase of data analysis was modeled on procedures put forth by van Kaam (1969) and Colaizzi (1978). In brief, it involved the following steps: transcribing, sifting through, and broadly classifying the verbatim data; transforming similar ideas into specific, discernible categories; and then recursively reapplying the established categories to additional interview data, to determine if the categories were relevant, necessary, and sufficient in capturing the totality of the data.

This process led to the ten HIV representations presented in Chapter 3. The representations are listed here, in order of the frequency with which they were mentioned by different participants. Numbers in parentheses indicate how many participants, and what percentage of the total N, mentioned each specific representation:

Representation	Number of Subjects Using Representation (Total $N = 19$)
1. HIV as Catalyst for Personal Growth	(14; 74%)
2. HIV as Belonging	(14; 74%)
3. HIV as Irreparable Loss	(14; 74%)
4. HIV as Punishment	(13; 68%)
5. HIV as a Contamination of One's Self	(11; 58%)
6. HIV as Strategy	(9; 47%)
7. HIV as Catalyst for Spiritual Growth	(8; 42%)
8. HIV as Isolation	(7; 37%)
9. HIV as Confirmation of Powerlessness	(6; 32%)
10. HIV as Relief	(4; 21%)

The second phase of data analysis explored a broader question: How did the men integrate HIV and AIDS into a more encompassing, coherent framework for reascribing meaning to life? Here again, categories were determined as they emerged from the data, rather than *a priori*, and recursively applied back to remaining data to determine their relevance and sufficiency. However, in addition to examining isolated verbatim quotes, other factors were now also taken into consideration: the men's affective presentation; the consistency of the material they reported; their primary defense mechanisms (as per Vaillant, 1986); and recurrent themes that developed within the course of each interview.

Four general patterns emerged. These patterns form the basis (also influenced by ongoing clinical work) of the styles of Transformation, Rupture, Camouflage, and Impassivity, described in Chapters 4 through 7. Among the participants, seven fit into the style I now call Transformation; four men fit into each of the other three patterns.

Limitations of the Study

The open-ended and exploratory nature of the study allowed for a great deal of rich clinical material and in-depth examination of each participant's unique experience. But because the study design (1) was cross-sectional rather than longitudinal; (2) did not randomize or compare subjects; and (3) employed relatively few "controls," it cannot lead to any causal conclusions. Further, 19 men is too small a sample from which to extrapolate into a broader population—if generalizations can ever accurately be made about such amorphous concepts as the "gay community" at all. And the study participants were by no means representative of the world at large: the sample was skewed in the direction of white, educated, economically stable men.

This study must also contend with a basic methodological concern that bedevils all research with self-selected populations: Who participates, and why? Although the breadth of responses among the men suggests that they chose to participate for a variety of reasons, the fact remains that these men elected to participate whereas many others did not, and that self-selection may influence the study's outcome.

Despite these limitations, it is hoped that this exploration of how HIV-positive gay men ascribe meaning to HIV and AIDS fills a gap in our knowledge about the psychosocial functioning of HIV-positive gay men in this crisis. The study is offered as a descriptive investigation of people's attempts to forge meaning in a medical epidemic and psychological crisis. It may serve as a springboard for other creative and detailed examinations of this crucial aspect of life amid AIDS.

Notes

Preface

1. From "Dirge without Music." In *Collected poems: Edna St. Vincent Millay.* (1956). New York: Harper & Row.

Chapter 1. A Crisis of Meaning

1. The Centers for Disease Control first mentioned an AIDS-related phenomenon in their weekly infectious disease newsletter, *Morbidity and Mortality Weekly Report (MMWR)*, on June 5, 1981 (*30, 21*). The next mention was July 3, 1981 (*30, 25*). By the end of May 1982, 355 cases of this still unnamed entity had been reported (*31, 22*), a few retroactively from the late 1970s. By December 1982, over 1,000 cases were reported (*MMWR Annual Survey*, 1982; *32, 54*). The CDC adopted and first used the term AIDS, for Acquired Immune Deficiency Syndrome, in September 1982 (*31, 37*).

2. One study participant, Anthony, knew of his immune impairment since December 1981, long before the actual discovery of HIV.

3. The length of time between infection and onset of symptoms varies greatly from person to person. A small percentage of HIV-positive individuals develop AIDS within a few years of infection; the majority develop AIDS within 15 years (Buchbinder, Katz, Hessol, O'Malley, & Holmberg, 1994; Kalichman, 1995). Several researchers report that seven to ten years typically elapse between the time of infection and onset of first symptoms (e.g., Friedman et al., 1991; Mills & Masur, 1990; Moss & Bacchetti, 1989). Despite this long period without major outward manifes-

tation of impairment, it now appears that the destructive progression of the virus can be strong from the time of infection on.

4. For reasons that remain uncertain, the length of time between infection and symptoms, and overall survival time, differ based on a person's age, gender, ethnicity, and means of infection (see Kalichman, 1995). It is generally assumed that a variety of potential cofactors influence the progression of the virus. As more research accrues, it seems that biological factors may play a role in this diversity (particularly with the issue of age). However, cultural factors (such as poverty, access to health care, and a long period of ignorance regarding HIV's impact in women) seem to be of greater influence in explaining survival differences. In fact, when timely access to health care and appropriate medical intervention are taken into account, inter-*group* differences of survival time diminish, while the inter-*individual* variability remains high (K. Mayer, personal communication, 1995).

5. For discussions of AIDS-related stigma, see Herek and Capitanio (1993); Herek and Glunt (1988); and Peters, den-Boer, Kok, and Schaalma (1994). A classic, influential exploration of the general topic of stigma is E. Goffman's *Stigma: Notes on the management of spoiled identity.* (1963). Englewood Cliffs, NJ: Prentice Hall.

6. I am alluding to the title of *Therapists on the front line: Psychotherapy with gay men in the age of AIDS* (Cadwell, Burnham, and Forstein 1994), a comprehensive edited volume dealing with psychotherapy of gay men who are seropositive, negative, or unsure of their HIV status.

Chapter 2. Meaning: The Perennial Quest

1. Baumeister (1991).

2. Janoff-Bulman (1992). For the purposes of my work, I highlight only one aspect of Dr. Janoff-Bulman's theory of peoples' underlying assumptions regarding life and the world. In addition to the meaning-related beliefs I focus on, Janoff-Bulman also contends that, in Western cultures, most non-traumatized individuals also hold key beliefs regarding the benevolence of the world and the worthiness of the self—beliefs that are equally subject to disruption in trauma or victimization.

3. Lerner (1980).

4. Langer (1975).

5. Langer & Roth (1975).

6. Kahneman, Slovic, and Tversky (1982).

7. Lerner (1980).

8. Farmer and Kleinman (1989) place "blaming the victim" within the context of a social milieu that regards autonomy and individual rights as supreme values. They contrast societal treatment of people with AIDS in America and Haiti. In America, a distinction is made between "innocent" AIDS victims, such as children, hemophiliacs, and recipients of HIV-infected blood transfusions, and, by inference, "guilty" victims—gay men, IV drug users and their partners, and prostitutes. By contrast, in Haiti, a culture where "individual rights are often underemphasized and also frequently unprotected" (Farmer & Kleinman, 1989, p. 146), individuals are held less accountable for their actions, and blaming the victim is not a response to people with AIDS.

9. Taylor (1989) presents a wealth of empirical evidence in support of her thesis. It is worth noting that the value of illusory self-deception was also understood by early psychoanalytic theorists, such as Otto Rank: "[A healthy person] can . . . repress, displace, deny, rationalize, or dramatize himself and deceive others. . . . [The neurotic] suffers . . . in the refusal of these mechanisms, which . . . robs him of the illusions important for living" (Rank, 1945, p. 251).

10. Frankl (1959).

11. *Ibid.*, p. 35

12. *Ibid.*, p. 95

13. *Ibid.*, p. 49

14. *Ibid.*, p. 75. Frankl states that he borrows this quotation from Dostoevski.

15. *Ibid.*, p. 47

16. Dimsdale (1980).

17. See, e.g., Lifton (1980).

18. *Ibid.*

19. *Ibid.*, p. 118

20. Lifton (1968).

21. Approximately 10% of infected individuals remain asymptomatic 15 years after infection (Buchbinder et al., 1994). Obviously, determining why certain people become long-term non-progressors is an area of important, active research.

22. See, e.g.,: Broyard (1992), Cousins (1979), Kushner (1975).

23. Kleinman (1988), p. xiii.

24. Viney, Henry, Walker, & Crooks (1989).

25. Hamera and Shontz (1978).

26. Susan Sontag's two relevant books are *Illness as metaphor* (1978) and *AIDS and its metaphors* (1989). In *AIDS and its metaphors*, Sontag concisely describes the cultural milieu that proved so unfortunately hospitable to HIV: "The view that sexually transmitted diseases are not serious reached its apogee in the 1970s, which was also when many male homosexuals reconstituted themselves as something like an ethnic group, one whose distinctive folkloric custom was sexual voracity, and the institutions of urban homosexual life became a sexual delivery system of unprecedented speed, efficiency and volume" (p.76).

27. White (1980), p. 16.

28. Over the past 20 years, many psychological models have been presented to describe the process of adopting a self-affirming gay or lesbian identity (see, e.g., Cass, 1979; Coleman, 1981–1982; Malyon, 1982; Troiden, 1979; Weinberg, 1983). Many writers from other disciplines have analyzed the emergence and development of the modern gay subculture from historical and sociological perspectives, pre-AIDS and current (see, e.g., Altman, 1982; Bersani, 1995; Bronski, 1984; Browning, 1993; Rofes, 1995). Explorations of the unprecedented phenomenon of the 1970s urban gay subculture tend to view gay men's emphasis on pleasure as a reaction against the sense of concealment and oppression that has long characterized society's attitudes toward homosexuality.

29. Kalichman (1995) provides a good review and discussion of HIV-related psychoneuroimmunological research. A few researchers have found a relationship between particular psychosocial factors (such as an active coping style) and immune functioning (e.g., Goodkin et al., 1992). Unfortunately, most studies have been unable to demonstrate a clear-cut interaction between factors such as stress reduction, a positive attitude, or social support and sustained changes in immunity. Yet interestingly, the inverse seems to hold true as well—negative psychological states, such as depression or anxiety, have *not* been associated with the onset of symptoms (e.g., Perry et al., 1992). Given the limitations of current research methodology, it seems premature to reach a conclusion on this matter in any direction.

30. A good general introduction to Buddhism may be found in Ross (1980).

Chapter 3. Representations of HIV and AIDS

I. Lipowski (1970–1971) presented a similar conceptual scheme for individuals facing severe illness. He labeled eight general categories of illness meanings: illness as challenge, illness as enemy, illness as punishment, illness as weakness, illness as relief, illness as strategy, illness as irreparable loss or damage, and illness as value.

2. In the interviews that I conducted, 14 of the 19 men (74%) identified at least some beneficial component of being HIV-positive (see Schwartzberg, 1993). Viney et al. (1989) also report HIV-positive individuals deriving benefit from their situation. Reports of individuals who describe deriving benefits from HIV infection can amply be found in the popular media. Typical in this regard is a *New York Times* front-page story (1990, June 17) headlined "After AIDS diagnosis, some embrace life."

3. Among major psychological theories that guide modern psychotherapy practice, object-relations theory and self-psychology (both of which are derived from psychoanalytic principles), attachment theory (based on the works of John Bowlby), and self-in-relation theory (an interpersonal feminist theory of Jean Baker Miller, Irene Stiver, Judy Jordan, and Jan Surrey) are all grounded in the human need to relate to others.

4. Freud (1950) and Levine (1982).

5. Parsons (1951).

6. Sontag (1989) asserts that "considering illness as a punishment is the oldest idea of what causes illness" (p. 45).

Chapter 4. Transformation: A Journey of Growth

I. Before the name "Acquired Immune Deficiency Syndrome" came into regular usage in late 1982, the disease was sometimes called GRID— "Gay-Related Immune Disease," or, more simply, "gay cancer" or "gay plague."

2. Callen (1990), pp. 10–11.

3. For more discussion of "dysfunctional denial" see Janoff-Bulman (1989).

4. Lifton explores the importance of "symbolic immortality" in facing death, individually and in the context of massive death experiences. See Lifton (1977).

5. Kahana, Harel, and Kahana (1988).

6. Janoff-Bulman (1992).

Chapter 5. Rupture: The Shattering of Meaning

1. Stroebe and Stroebe (1987) provide a comprehensive analysis of the psychological literature on widowhood. Many factors likely influence the course of grief in widowhood. Support for the hypothesis that highly dependent or ambivalent relationships are most likely to predispose a widow for a prolonged grief reaction comes primarily from the investigations of Parkes and Weiss (1983) and Lopata (1979).

2. The most detailed investigation of AIDS-related bereavement has been a longitudinal epidemiological study of gay men in New York City, begun in 1984 by the late John Martin and his colleagues (e.g., Dean, 1995; Martin, 1988; Martin & Dean, 1993). For clinical discussions of AIDS-related grief, see Klein and Fletcher, 1986; Sherr, 1995; and Schwartzberg, 1992.

3. Horowitz (1976).

4. Puig (1991).

5. The line is from the song "It's alright ma (I'm only bleeding)." Dylan, B. (1985).

6. The topic of resilience is an area of much psychological research. Many of these studies focus on children who face extreme stressors—those born into poverty or families where alcoholism, violence, abuse, or severe mental illness is present (see Luthar & Zigler, 1991, for a review). A few investigations have examined resilience in adults facing HIV (e.g., Rabkin, Remien, Katoff, & Williams, 1993; Schwartzberg, 1994).

7. The most comprehensive data on war-related trauma come from the National Vietnam Veterans Readjustment Study (NVVRS), a large-scale investigation mandated by Congress in 1983 to document the rates of PTSD and other types of psychological distress among veterans. A full account of the study is presented in Kulka et al. (1990).

Chapter 6. Camouflage: The Fine Line of Self-Deception

1. Most people tend to employ a *self-serving bias* (Miller & Ross, 1975) in how we view ourselves in the world: We are apt to attribute our successes to *internal* aspects of ourselves, but to discount our failures by

regarding them as caused by *external* features. We don't typically grant others the same leniency. Social psychologists have examined this bias in a multitude of ways.

2. Most of the men I interviewed likely contracted HIV early in the epidemic. Some probably had been infected as early as the 1970s. I interviewed Francis in 1990. When he referred to men who were infected by "free choice," he was nonetheless referring to the early confusing years of the epidemic, when knowledge was fuzzier or nonexistent about the HIV-related health risks of sex.

3. Fleishman (1989), pp. 152–153.

4. Not all defense mechanisms are equally adaptive. Several theorists (e.g., Perry & Cooper, 1986; Vaillant, 1986) have catalogued and ranked various defense mechanisms, looking at the extent to which they distort reality or interfere with interpersonal functioning. Vaillant (1986) proposes a hierarchy of four general levels of defensive/adaptive functioning: psychotic, immature, neurotic, and healthy. Among the men I interviewed, those with a Camouflage style of adaptation gave more examples of using immature and neurotic defense mechanisms; men with a style of Transformation tended to demonstrate more neurotic and healthy defenses.

5. Fleishman, *op cit.*

Chapter 7. Impassivity: Minimizing the Trauma

1. With then-current CDC diagnostic criteria, Sam did not have AIDS, because he had experienced no major opportunistic infection. With the diagnostic criteria the CDC put into effect in 1993, he would be considered a person with AIDS, because the newer description added a T-cell count below 200 as one of the criteria.

2. See Matt Fuller's essay in *The Advocate* (November 29, 1994) about his decision to tattoo the words "HIV-Positive" and a pink triangle on his arm. Tewksbury (1994) looks specifically at the language HIV-positive individuals use to describe themselves in the context of managing self-identity.

3. See Shapiro (1965); he discusses the circular relationship between how people perceive the world and then, based on these perceptions, interact with others. Shapiro theorizes that individuals with different character styles also have different styles of memory, because of what they attend to in the world, how they attend to it, and what they consider most salient.

4. Harris was referring to the American military involvement in the Persian Gulf War, which occurred shortly before our interview in April 1991.

5. Wortman and Silver (1989) explore what they label "the myths of coping." They maintain that many of our deepest cultural assumptions about how people deal with a traumatic loss are not necessarily true. Among the myths they question are: (1) depression is an inevitable consequence of loss; (2) absence of depression indicates a pathological response; and (3) all significant losses need to be "worked through" in order to be healed.

6. Downey, Silver, & Wortman (1990).

7. Several large-scale studies, such as the Multicenter AIDS Cohort Study (e.g., Ostrow et al., 1989; Lyketsos, Hoover et al., 1993) and the San Francisco Men's Health Study (Burrack et al., 1993), as well as many smaller ones have looked at gay men's psychological responses to HIV. Many HIV-positive individuals meet clinical criteria for depressive disorders, anxiety disorders, or post-traumatic stress disorder — but far fewer than early estimates had predicted (Kalichman, 1995). What emerges from many of these studies is the unexpected *lack* of major psychological impairment in many individuals (e.g., Kessler et al., 1988; King, 1989): "The results [of the MACS study] show clearly that a substantial percentage of the men in this cohort experience clinically significant emotional impairment. Yet, at the same time, it is striking to find that the vast majority have managed to maintain relatively normal emotional functioning despite the danger, loss and uncertainty which the AIDS epidemic entails" (Kessler et al., 1989, p. 573).

The most common psychological disorder for HIV-positive individuals seems to be Adjustment Disorder with depressed or anxious mood. This disorder is a depressed or anxious reaction that develops in response to a particularly stressor, lasts a brief time, and then remits, with a person returning to his or her previous level of functioning.

Chapter 8. Living with Uncertainty, Ambiguity, and Questions of Mortality

1. Ralph Waldo Emerson's actual words were, "A foolish consistency is the hobgoblin of little minds, adored by little statesmen, philosophers, and divines" (from *Essays, First Series*, 1841).

2. Even the points addressed as "scientific progress" are still marked by ambiguity and uncertainty. For example, regarding paths of transmission, it seems clear that certain sexual practices (such as receptive anal intercourse) place an individual at high risk for infection. Yet other practices, such as oral sex, with or without the transmission of semen and/or pre-seminal fluid, remain in a cloudy region of "possibly" risky. Cases of oral transmission of HIV have been documented, yet it also seems likely that this is a far less risky activity than anal sex. Safer sex guidelines vary from organization to organization and locale to locale, often with heated disagreements about how to classify these more ambiguous sexual practices.

Additionally, identifying HIV as the causal agent in AIDS is not without its critics (e.g., Duesberg, 1996), who maintain that HIV may be correlated with AIDS without causing it. And various strains of HIV have been identified (Gallo & Montagnier, 1988), although it seems likely that HIV-2 is less virulent than HIV-1 (Marlink et al., 1994).

3. For a discussion of the deleterious effects of these media distortions see: Callen (1990) and Watney (1988).

4. The relationship between hope and denial is explored by Janoff-Bulman and Timko (1987). They argue that hope can flower even (or particularly) in situations where the worst outcomes are imagined. The ability to maintain optimism even in the face of a traumatizing reality is a "protection that serves to shield us from experiencing utter misery and despair" Janoff-Bulman & Timko (1987), p.155.

5. Benjamin (1968), pp. 93–94.

6. Getzel and Mahoney (1990), p. 106.

Chapter 9. Coping, Changing, Growing

1. See, e.g., Lazarus and Folkman (1984) or Lazarus (1991).

2. Lazarus and Folkman, *ibid.*, p. 141.

3. Benner, Roskies, and Lazarus (1980).

4. Many books about coping with psychological distress appeal because they attempt to render comprehensible—and controllable—matters that may seem too large or overwhelming to tolerate. The work of Elizabeth Kubler-Ross on dying is a good example. In her 1969 book, *On Death and Dying*, Kubler-Ross broke important ground by humanely describing psychological reactions to facing one's own death. By extrapolation, her work has been applied to how people grieve the death of others. Her five-stage model of coping with death and dying—shock, denial,

anger, bargaining, and acceptance—has gained immense popularity, professionally and among the general public. In fact, at a mass level, this has become one of the most popularized nuggets of all modern psychological thought. It has been culturally codified as the expectable way to grieve.

Yet, despite its widespread popularity, the model does not, in fact, accurately describe how most people respond to loss (e.g., Lehman, Wortman, & Williams, 1987; Schwartzberg & Janoff-Bulman, 1991; Wortman & Silver, 1989; Zisook & Shuchter, 1986). Instead, grief seems to be a highly individual process, with significant interpersonal variability in the length, nature, and style of grieving. Studies of various bereaved populations fail to support the existence of a solitary, stage-model of grief.

So why does it remain so popular? In part, because applied in isolated pieces and not too rigidly, it likely approximates enough people's experiences so that they forgive or ignore the rest. But more than this, I suspect the model appeals because it fills our need to translate that which is mysterious and amorphous into something predictable, tractable, and orderly. How comforting to have a time-limited, five-stage process to explain the enigma of death.

Stage models of grief are particularly ill suited when applied to gay men's AIDS-related grief, given the reality of multiple, cumulative losses and the unique nature of grief in massive death experiences (see Lifton, 1968; Schwartzberg, 1992).

5. "No man is an island, entire of itself. . . ." John Donne, *Hymn to God My God, in my Sickness* (1623 or 1631).

6. *Schema theory* is a main concept in the psychological field of "social cognition." According to this theory (and well supported with research data), people hold organized collections of beliefs regarding themselves, others, social roles, and events. Incoming information that is consistent with our established schemata are more easily attended to, stored, and retrieved than information that contradicts these established patterns. See Fiske and Taylor (1984).

7. This is not meant to be a comprehensive list of compulsive behaviors. For example, in addition to the misuse of food, alcohol, drugs, and sex, compulsive gambling or spending can also interfere with appropriate coping.

8. Feinberg (1994), p. 135.

9. Lipowski (1970–1971); see also Mechanic (1966). This range of coping styles has important ramifications for medical patients. For some

individuals, hearing detailed descriptions of their physical situation or upcoming procedures will lessen their anxiety; for others, the details only add to their worry.

10. The Kabbalah is a school of Jewish mysticism dating back to the twelfth century. Its primary text is the Zohar. Similar paradoxical notions are expressed in other religions and philosophical systems, such as the ancient Chinese concept of yin and yang, or the Hindu goddess Kali, who both lovingly creates and vengefully destroys. The ancient Greek philosopher Heraclitus elaborated a notion of *enantiodromia*, the interdependence of opposites, which was adopted by Carl Jung: "Every psychological extreme secretly contains its own opposite or stands in some sort of intimate and essential relation to it ... the more extreme a position is, the more easily we may expect an enantiodromia" (Jung, 1952, p. 375).

Chapter 10. Grief and Hope

1. The concept of "emotional truth" can also be taken too far. For example, we enter dangerous waters when we assume that all emotional pain points in the direction of a history of abuse. I reject current formulations of life difficulties that follow the prescription, "If you think you were abused, you probably were." While we know now that childhood abuse (physical, sexual, and emotional) is distressingly common, with harmful and long-lasting psychological aftereffects, it is still important to exercise caution in jumping from the complex world of emotional and unconscious phenomena to the assumption of actual abuse.

2. Wilder (1986), p. 139.

3. Empirical data support the importance of ascribing meaning in adversity. The need to reestablish the belief in a meaningful and safe world has been found among people who have experienced terminal illness, the death of a parent or child, the loss of a limb, rape, and personal assault (Janoff-Bulman, 1989; Lehman et al., 1987; Schwartzberg & Janoff-Bulman, 1991; Wortman & Silver, 1987, 1989; see also Funk, 1992, and Kobasa, 1979, on psychological "hardiness," or the psychoneuroimmunological benefits of feeling a sense of commitment in life).

Given this support, and the common-sense appeal of the topic, the question arises: Why has such a fundamental aspect of dealing with adversity received such relatively sparse attention? The answer may have more to do with the peculiarities of academic scientific research than with a rejection of the topic. Inquiries into meaningfulness fall between the cracks of various disciplines. For most current academic psychologists, the questions are too open-ended and exploratory. They don't lend themselves well to numerical or objective study. However, for disciplines such as sociology or cultural anthropology, such questions are too clinically specific. They examine individual differences, and intrapsychic dynamics, rather than group trends.

4. Stall, Coates, and Hoff (1988).

5. Allport (1980).

6. The words are those of the Rev. Dr. Kenneth Orth, from a homily preached at an AIDS Healing Service in 1994.

References

Allport, G. (1980). *The nature of prejudice*. Reading, MA: Addison-Wesley. (Originally published in 1954.)

Altman, D. (1982). *The homosexualization of America, the Americanization of the homosexual*. New York: St. Martin's Press.

Baumeister, R. F. (1991). *Meanings of life*. New York: Guilford.

Benjamin, W. (1968). *Illuminations: Essays and reflections*. New York: Schocken.

Benner, P., Roskies, E., & Lazarus, R. S. (1980). Stress and coping under extreme in conditions. In J. E. Dimsdale, ed., *Survivors, victims, and perpetrators: Essays on the Nazi holocaust*. Washington, DC: Hemisphere.

Bersani, L. (1995). *Homos*. Cambridge, MA: Harvard University Press.

Bronski, M. (1984). *Culture clash: The making of gay sensibility*. Boston: South End Press.

Browning, F. (1993). *The culture of desire: Paradox and perversity in gay lives today*. New York: Vintage.

Broyard, A. (1992). *Intoxicated by my illness*. New York: Fawcett Columbine.

Buchbinder, S. P., Katz, M. H., Hessol, N. A., O'Malley, P. M., & Holmberg, S. D. (1994). Long-term HIV-I infection without immunologic progression. *AIDS. 8, 8,* 1123–1128.

Burrack, J. H., Barrett, D. C., Stall, R., Chesney, M. A., Ekstrand, M. L., & Coates, T. J. (1993). Depressive symptoms and CD4 lymphocyte decline among HIV-infected men. *Journal of the American Medical Association, 270,* 2568–2573.

Cadwell, S. A., Burnham, R. A., & Forstein, M., eds. (1994). *Therapists on the front line: Psychotherapy with gay men in the age of AIDS*. Washington, DC: American Psychiatric Press.

Callen, M. (1990). *Surviving AIDS.* New York: HarperCollins.

Cass, V. (1979). Homosexual identity formation. *Journal of Homosexuality, 4* (3), 219–235.

Centers for Disease Control. (1981). *Morbidity and Mortality Weekly Report, 30, 21.*

Centers for Disease Control. (1981). *Morbidity and Mortality Weekly Report, 30, 25.*

Centers for Disease Control. (1982). *Morbidity and Mortality Weekly Report, 31, 22.*

Centers for Disease Control. (1982). *Morbidity and Mortality Weekly Report, 31, 37.*

Centers for Disease Control. (1983). *Morbidity and Mortality Weekly Report, Annual Survey, 1982, 32, 54.*

Centers for Disease Control. (1986). Classification systems for human T-lymphotropic virus: Type III/lymphadenopathy associated virus infections. *Morbidity and Mortality Weekly Report, 35,* 334–339.

Centers for Disease Control. (1987). Revision of the case definition of acquired immunodeficiency syndrome for national reporting—United States. *Morbidity and Mortality Weekly Report, 36, 15.*

Centers for Disease Control. (1991). *HIV—AIDS Surveillance Report* (May 1991).

Colaizzi, P. F. (1978). Psychological research as the phenomenologist views it. In R. S. Valle & M. King, eds., *Existential-phenomenological alternatives for psychology.* New York: Oxford University Press.

Coleman, E. (1981–1982). Developmental stages of the coming out process. *Journal of homosexuality, 7* (2–3).

Cousins, N. (1979). *Anatomy of an illness as perceived by the patient: Reflections on healing and regeneration.* New York: Norton.

Dean, L. (1995). The epidemiology and impact of AIDS-related death and dying in New York's gay community. In L. Sherr, ed., *Grief and AIDS.* Chichester, England: John Wiley & Sons.

Dimsdale, J. E. (1980). The coping behavior of Nazi concentration camp survivors. In J. E. Dimsdale, ed., *Survivors, victims, and perpetrators: Essays on the Nazi holocaust.* Washington, DC: Hemisphere.

Downey, G., Silver, R. C., & Wortman, C. B. (1990). Reconsidering the attribution-adjustment relation following a major negative event: Coping with the loss of a child. *Journal of Personality and Social Psychology 59, 5,* 925–940.

Duesberg, P. (1996). *Inventing the AIDS virus.* Washington, D.C.: Regnery.

Dylan, B. (1985). *Lyrics, 1962–1985.* New York: Knopf.

Farmer, P., & Kleinman, A. (1989). AIDS as human suffering. *Daedelus (Journal of the American Academy of Arts and Sciences), 118*(2), 135–160.

Feinberg, D. (1994). *Queer and loathing: Rants and raves of a raging AIDS clone.* New York: Viking.

Fiske, S. T., & Taylor, S. E. (1984). *Social cognition.* Reading, MA: Addison-Wesley.

Fleischman, P. R. (1989). *The healing spirit: Explorations in religion and psychotherapy.* New York: Paragon House.

Frankl, V. (1959). *Man's search for meaning.* Boston: Beacon Press. (Originally published 1946.)

Freud, S. (1950). *Beyond the pleasure principle.* New York: Liveright. (Originally published 1920.)

Friedman, Y., Franklin, C., Freels, S., & Weil, M. H. (1991). Long-term survival of patients with AIDS, *Pneumocystis carinii* pneumonia, and respiratory failure. *Journal of the American Medical Association, 266,* 89–92.

Fuller, M. (1994, November 29). Marked man. *The Advocate,* p. 6.

Funk, S. C. (1992). Hardiness: A review of theory and research. *Health Psychology, 11, 5,* 335–345.

Gallo, R. C. & Montagnier, L. (1988). AIDS in 1988. *Scientific American, 259,* 41–48.

Getzel, G. S., & Mahoney, K. (1990). Confronting human finitude: Group work with people with AIDS. *Journal of Gay and Lesbian Psychotherapy, 1, 3,* 105–120.

Giorgi, A. (1985). *Phenomenology and psychological research.* Pittsburgh: Duquesne University Press.

Goffman, E. (1963). *Stigma: Notes on the management of spoiled identity.* Englewood, Cliffs, NJ: Prentice-Hall.

Goodkin, K., Blaney, N. T., Feaster, D., Fletcher, M. A., Baum, M. K., Atienza, E. M., Klimas, N. G., Millon, C., Szapocznik, J., & Eisdorfer, C. (1992). Active coping style is associated with natural killer cell cytotoxicity in asymptomatic HIV-1 seropositive homosexual men. *Journal of Psychosomatic Research, 36,* 635–650.

Hall, T. (1990, June 17). After AIDS diagnosis, some embrace life. *The New York Times,* pp. 1, 20.

Hamera, E. K., & Shontz, F. (1978). Perceived positive and negative effects of life-threatening illness. *Journal of Psychosomatic Research, 22,* 419–424.

Herek, G. M., & Capitanio, J. P. (1993). Public reactions to AIDS in the United States: A second decade of stigma. *American Journal of Public Health, 83, 4,* 574–577.

Horowitz, M. (1976). *Stress response syndromes.* New York: Aronson.

Janoff-Bulman, R. (1989). The benefits of illusions, the threat of disillusionment, and the limitations of inaccuracy. *Journal of Social and Clinical Psychology, 8,* 158–175.

Janoff-Bulman, R. (1992). *Shattered assumptions: Towards a new psychology of trauma.* New York: Free Press.

Janoff-Bulman, R., & Timko, C. (1987). Coping with traumatic life events: The role of denial in light of people's assumptive worlds. In C. R. Snyder and C. Ford, eds., *Coping with negative life events: Clinical and social perspectives.* New York: Plenum.

Jung, C. G. (1952). *Symbols of transformation.* New York: Bollingen Foundation.

Kahana, B., Harel, A., & Kahana, E. (1988). Predictors of psychological well-being among survivors of the Holocaust. In J. P. Wilson, Z. Harel, & B. Kahana, eds., *Human adaptation to extreme stress: From the Holocaust to Vietnam.* New York: Plenum.

Kahneman, D., Slovic, P., & Tversky, A., eds. (1982). *Judgment under uncertainty: Heuristics and biases.* Englewood Cliffs, NJ: Prentice-Hall.

Kalichman, S. (1995). *Understanding AIDS: A guide for mental health professionals.* Washington, DC: American Psychological Association.

Kessler, R. C., O'Brien, K., Joseph, J. G., Ostrow, D. G., Phair, J. P., Chmiel, J. S., Wortman, C. B., & Emmons, C. (1988). Effects of HIV infection, perceived health and clinical status on a cohort at risk for AIDS. *Social Science and Medicine, 27*(6), 569–578.

King, M. B. (1989). Psychosocial status of 192 outpatients with HIV infection and AIDS. *British Journal of Psychiatry, 154,* 237–242.

Klein, S. J., & Fletcher, W. (1986). Gay grief: An examination of its uniqueness brought to light by the AIDS crisis. *Journal of Psychosocial Oncology, 4,* 15–25.

Kleinman, A. (1988). *The illness narratives: Suffering, healing, and the human condition.* New York: Basic Books.

Kobasa, S. C. (1979). Stressful life events, personality and health: An inquiry into hardiness. *Journal of Personality and Social Psychology 37*, I–II.

Kubler-Ross, E. (1969). *On death and dying.* New York: Macmillan.

Kulka, R. A., Schlenger, W. E., Fairbank, J. A., Hough, R. S., Jordan, B. K., Marmar, C. R., & Weiss, D. S. (1990). *Trauma and the Vietnam War generation: Report of findings from the National Vietnam Veterans Readjustment Study.* New York: Brunner/Mazel.

Kushner, R. (1975). *Why Me?* New York: New American Library.

Langer, E. J. (1975). The illusion of control. *Journal of Personality and Social Psychology, 32,* 311–328.

Langer, E. J., & Roth, J. (1975). Heads I win, tails it's chance: The illusion of control as a function of the sequence outcomes in a purely chance event. *Journal of Personality Social Psychology, 32,* 951–955.

Lazarus, R. S. (1991). *Emotion and adaptation.* New York: Oxford University Press.

Lazarus, R. S., & Folkman, S. (1984). *Stress, appraisal, and coping.* New York: Springer.

Lehman, D. R., Wortman, C. B., & Williams, A. F. (1987). Long-term effects of losing a spouse or child in a motor vehicle crash. *Journal of Personality and Social Psychology, 52 (1),* 218–231.

Lerner, M. J. (1980). *The belief in a just world: A fundamental delusion.* New York: Plenum.

Levine, S. (1982). *Who dies? An investigation of conscious living and conscious dying.* New York: Anchor.

Lifton, R. J. (1968). *Death in life: Survivors of Hiroshima.* New York: Random House.

Lifton, R. J. (1977). The sense of immortality: On death and the continuation of life. In H. Feifel, ed., *New meanings of death.* New York: McGraw-Hill.

Lifton, R. J. (1980). The concept of the survivor. In J. E. Dimsdale, ed., *Survivors, victims, and perpetrators: Essays on the Nazi holocaust.* Washington, DC: Hemisphere.

Lipowski, Z. J. (1970–1971). Physical illness, the individual and the coping process. *International Journal of Psychiatry in Medicine, 1,* 91–102.

Lopata, H. Z. (1979). *Women as widows: Support systems.* New York: Elsevier.

Luthar, S. S., & Zigler, E. (1991). Vulnerability and competence: A review of research on resilience in childhood. *American Journal of Ortho-psychiatry, 61, 1,* 6–22.

Lyketsos, C. C. G., Hoover, D., Guccione, M., Senterfitt, W., Dew, A., Wesch, J., VanRaden, M., Treisman, G., & Morgenstern, H. (1993). Depressive symptoms as predictors of medical outcomes in HIV infection. *Journal of the American Medical Association, 270,* 2563–2567.

Malyon, A. K. (1982). Biphasic aspects of homosexual identity formation: Coming out as a second adolescence. *Psychotherapy, 19*(3), 335–340.

Marlink, R., Kanki, P., Thior, I., Travers, K., Eisen, G., Siby, T., Traore, I., Hsieh, C. C., Dia, M. C., Gueye, E. H. (1994). Reduced rate of disease development after HIV-2 infection as compared to HIV-I. *Science, 265,* 1587–1590.

Martin, J. L. (1988). Psychological consequences of AIDS-related bereavement among gay men. *Journal of Consulting and Clinical Psychology, 56, 6,* 856–862.

Martin, J. L., & Dean. L. (1993). Effects of AIDS-related bereavement and HIV-related illness on psychological distress among gay men: A 7-year longitudinal study, 1985–1991. *Journal of Consulting and Clinical Psychology, 61,* 94–103,

Mechanic, D. (1966). Response factors in illness: The study of illness behavior. *Social Psychiatry, 1,* 11–20.

Millay, E. St. Vincent (1956). Dirge without music. In *Collected poems: Edna St. Vincent Millay.* New York: Harper & Row.

Miller, D. T., & Ross, M. (1975). Self-serving biases in the attribution of causality: Fact or fiction? *Psychology Bulletin, 82,* 213–225.

Mills, J., & Masur, H. (1990). AIDS-related infections. *Scientific American, 263*(2), 50–57.

Milosz, C. (1993). The thistle, the nettle. In *Provinces: Poems, 1987–1991.* New York: Norton.

Moss, A. R., & Bacchetti, P. (1989). Natural history of HIV infection. *AIDS, 3,* 55–61.

Ostrow, D. G., Monjan, A., Joseph, J., VanRaden, M., Fox, R., Kingsley, L., Dudley, J., & Phair, J. (1989). HIV-related symptoms and psychological functioning in a cohort of homosexual men. *American Journal of Psychiatry, 146*(6), 737–742.

Parkes, C. M. (1988). Bereavement as a psychosocial transition: Process of adaptation to change. *Journal of Social Issues, 44*(3), 53–66.

Parkes, C. M., & Weiss, R. S. (1983). *Recovery from bereavement.* New York: Basic Books.

Parsons, T. (1951). *The social system.* Glencoe, IL: Free Press.

Perry, J. C., & Cooper, S. H. (1986). What do cross-sectional measures of defense mechanisms predict? In G. Vaillant, ed., *Empirical studies of ego mechanisms of defense.* Washington, DC: American Psychiatric Press.

Perry, S., Fishman, B., Jacobsberg, L., & Frances, A. (1992), Relationships over 1 year between lymphocyte subsets and psychosocial variables among adults with infection by human immunodeficiency virus. *Archives of General Psychiatry, 49,* 396–401.

Peters, L., den-Boer, D. J., Kok, G., & Schaalma, H. P. (1994). Public reactions towards people with AIDS: An attributional analysis. *Patient Education and Counseling, 24,* 3, 323–335.

Polkinghorne, D. E. (1989). Phenomenological research methods. In R. S. Valle & S. Halling, eds., *Existential-phenomenological perspectives in psychology: Exploring the breadth of human experience.* New York: Plenum.

Puig, M. (1991). *Kiss of the spiderwoman.* New York: International Vintage. (Originally published 1978.)

Rabkin, J. G., Remien, R., Katoff, L., & Williams, J. B. (1993). Resilience in adversity among long-term survivors of AIDS. *Hospital and Community Psychiatry, 44,* 2, 162–167.

Rank, O. (1945). *Will therapy and truth and reality.* New York: Knopf.

Rofes, E. (1995). *Reviving the tribe: Regenerating gay men's sexuality and culture in the ongoing epidemic.* New York: Harrington Park Press.

Ross, N. W. (1980). *Buddhism: A way of life and thought.* New York: Vintage.

Schwartzberg, S. (1992). AIDS-related bereavement among gay men: The inadequacy of current theories of grief. *Psychotherapy, 29,* 3, 422–429.

Schwartzberg, S. (1993). Struggling for meaning: How HIV-positive gay men make sense of AIDS. *Professional Psychology: Research and Practice, 24,* 4, 483–490.

Schwartzberg, S. (1994). Vitality and growth in HIV-infected gay men. *Social Science and Medicine, 38,* 4, 593–602.

Schwartzberg, S., & Janoff-Bulman, R. (1991). Exploring the assumptive worlds of bereaved college students: Grief and the search for meaning. *Journal of Social and Clinical Psychology, 10,* 3, 270–278.

Shapiro, D. (1965). *Neurotic styles.* New York: Basic Books.

Sherr, L. (Ed.). 1995. *Grief and AIDS*. Chichester, England: John Wiley & Sons.

Sontag, S. (1978). *Illness as metaphor*. New York: Farrar, Straus and Giroux.

Sontag, S. (1989). *AIDS and its metaphors*. New York: Farrar, Straus and Giroux.

Stall, R. D., Coates, T. J., & Hoff, C. (1988). Behavioral risk reduction for HIV infection among gay and bisexual men: A review of results from the United States. *American Psychologist, 43, 11*, 878–885.

Stroebe, W., & Stroebe, M. S. (1987). *Bereavement and health: The psychological and physical consequences of partner loss*. Cambridge: Cambridge University Press.

Taylor, S. E. (1989). *Positive illusions: Creative self-deception and the healthy mind*. New York: Basic Books.

Tewksbury, R. (1994). "Speaking of someone with AIDS . . . ": Identity constructions of persons with HIV disease. *Deviant Behavior, 15, 4*, 337–355.

Troiden, R. (1979). Becoming homosexual: A model of gay identity acquisition. *Psychiatry 42*, 362–373.

Vaillant, G. E. (Ed.). (1986). *Empirical studies of ego mechanisms of defense*. Washington, DC: American Psychiatric Press.

van Kaam, A. (1969). *Existential foundation of psychology*. New York: Image Books. (Originally published 1966.)

Viney, L. L., Henry, R., Walker, B. M., & Crooks, L. (1989). The emotional reactions of HIV antibody positive men. *British Journal of Medical Psychology, 62, 2*, 153–161.

Watney, S. (1988). The spectacle of AIDS. In D. Crimp, ed., *AIDS: Cultural analysis, cultural activism*. Cambridge, MA: MIT Press.

Weinberg, T. S. (1983). *Gay men, gay selves: The social construction of homosexual identities*. New York: Irvington.

White, E. (1980). *States of desire: Travels in gay America*. New York: E. P. Dutton.

Wilder, T. (1986). *Bridge of San Luis Rey*. New York: Harper & Row. (Originally published 1927.)

Wortman, C. B., & Silver, R. C. (1989). The myths of coping. *Journal of Consulting and Clinical Psychology, 57*, 349–357.

Zisook, S., & Shuchter, S. (1986). The first four years of widowhood. *Psychiatric Annals, 16*, 288–294

Index